PRAISE FOR *Electrical Nutrition*

"Denie Hiestand's revolutionary approach looks at why we as a society have developed so many diseases and illnesses. He takes the reader beyond normal perceived interpretations and deep into the electrical causes behind the physical manifestations. Denie shares unique hypotheses about the body, why it stops working and how to help it back onto its healing path. He offers the reader profound insights into their own lives and challenges everyone to reassess their approach to eating and being. His simple yet seemingly extreme suggestions concerning diet and supplementation from an electrical viewpoint will shake you up and rattle your ideas."
—*Townsend Letter for Doctors and Patients*

"A book full of 'shocking' news. Gives readers provocative thoughts about our bodies and nourishment that could set a new standard for the new era. . . . Astonishing stuff."

—*The Book Reader*

"*Electrical Nutrition* is a practical self-help health book which will stimulate and challenge many belief structures, but if put to the test will drastically improve health and vitality. Not only does it cover nutritional information, but is also food for the body, heart, and soul.

"Powerful, dynamic, and controversial, the authors take an electrical/energy perspective on everything from understanding ourselves, our bodies, and our world, to alleviating disease and formulating our supplements and medicine."
—*Leading Edge Review*

"If you think you've heard all the pros and cons of becoming a vegetarian, *Electrical Nutrition* will make you think again."

—*Shared Vision*

Nutrition

A Revolutionary
Approach to Eating
That Awakens the
Body's Natural
Electrical Energy

Most Avery books are available at special quantity discounts for bulk purchase for sales promotions, premiums, fund-raising, and educational needs. Special books or book excerpts also can be created to fit specific needs. For details, write Putnam Special Markets, 375 Hudson Street, New York, NY 10014.

a member of
Penguin Group (USA) Inc.
375 Hudson Street
New York, NY 10014
www.penguin.com

Library of Congress Cataloging-in-Publication Data

Hiestand, Denie.
    Electrical nutrition : a revolutionary approach to eating that awakens the body's
natural electrical energy / Denie Hiestand and Shelley Hiestand.
        p.   cm.
    Includes bibliographical references and index.
    ISBN 1-58333-106-9
    1. Alternative medicine.   2. Nutrition—Miscellanea.   I. Hiestand, Shelley.   II. Title.
R733.H54   2001   2001040192
613.2—dc21

Printed in the United States of America
10   9   8   7

Book design by Lee Fukui

To Frank Reglin and Mel and Kathy Tarry for having the vision and strength to follow your truth. To all the thousands of clients I have seen over the years who have allowed me to put my theories into practice and enabled me to learn and understand the truth of my own convictions. For this I thank you. And to Shelley, for your unwavering love and your passion for life that is my inspiration. Thank you, my love.

—DENIE

I would like to dedicate this edition to my father, one of the most inspirational, heart-centered, dedicated men on this planet, who died suddenly in 1999 of clogged arteries, nine years after he had six major bypasses and twenty-seven years after his first heart attack. I wish he had understood earlier the power and wisdom of *electrical nutrition*. Fitness and the recommended Heart Foundation diet didn't work in his case. If only he had listened to Denie, perhaps he would still be alive today. May *Electrical Nutrition* be an inspiration to all of humanity, to see beyond the falsehoods and misinformation so prevalent in today's world and realize the truth of these words. Denie has the ability to tell it how it really is with a simplicity and clarity so hard to find. His passion keeps my own fire burning and inspires me to share my light and joy with everyone. Thank you, Denie, for your love and a togetherness that people search lifetimes for that we have rediscovered and are now able to allow to flow in our life's work. I am eternally grateful for this wonderful gift called life.

—SHELLEY

Contents

Acknowledgments

A special thank you to John Gray, Ph.D., for his wonderful support of the work that we do. We are eternally grateful and blessed to know you.

Thanks go to Dr. Stephen Vizzard, Ph.D., P.S., Bellevue, Washington; Dr. Kim Kimball, M.D., Everett, Washington; Dr. Keith Mumby, Ph.D., Manchester, England; Peter Baumann, Ph.D., Bern, Switzerland; Dr. Linda C. Hole, M.D., Spokane, Washington; Dr. Paula Baruffi, N.D., Bellevue, Washington; Dr. Alex Mazurin, N.D., Penticton, British Columbia; and Dr. David Elliot for his book *Electrical Universe*—when I read this book I yelled out with glee, "There is somebody else who understands!"

Thank you also to all the other medical people with whom I have worked over the last fifteen years and who have had the patience to withstand my unceasing questions and to be willing, and sometimes not-so-willing, friendly adversaries in passionate debates about the way the body works. I would especially like to thank Judy Kubrak, for her incredible medical research information, and Robert Kalan, who generously contributed his editing skills to our self-published first edition. And to the thousands of authors whose names I may have forgotten over the years whose insights have allowed me to piece together my own theories. Without all the work that has preceded me and all the knowledge that is already in existence, I would not be able to share my knowing. Thank you also to the editors at Penguin Putnam who helped organize this book's contents: Laura Shepherd, Amy Tecklenburg, and Dara Stewart.

Foreword by John Gray

Many people search for fulfillment and happiness in their lives—alone and with a partner. Denie and Shelley are two people who live and breathe vitality and aliveness. This book offers practical, insightful information about how we can all gain more health and vitality.

I have personally been interested in health and healing for many years, and it has been refreshing to meet Denie and Shelley and become familiar with their work. They take an unapologetic stance and have the courage to state many things that challenge commonly accepted beliefs. Blatant though the book can be, in it Denie explains a truth from an energy perspective that very few people perceive. He takes what could be called *medical intuitiveness* straight into the realms of full conscious reality. He walks a fine line somewhere between being overly provocative and genuinely concerned about the future of humanity's health.

This book will certainly wake people up and get them thinking about what is real and what is true for them. Denie's down-to-earth logic is undeniable. He explains his seemingly outrageous concepts in a very realistic, accessible way so that no confusion remains. He offers a lot of practical suggestions for what people can do on a daily basis to increase their energy levels and get more out of life. Once you are happy with your own health, it is a lot easier to attract what you want into your life.

Denie and Shelley embody *Electrical Nutrition*. They are full of health and vitality and make the most of every opportunity, enjoying every experience. It is a blessing to know them both. I highly recommend *Electrical Nutrition* to anyone interested in pursuing vibrant health and happiness. It may rock your foundations, but sometimes that's a good thing. Read it and see for yourself.

—JOHN GRAY, PH.D., author of
Men Are from Mars, Women Are from Venus

Foreword by Robert Kalan

I sing the body electric,
The armies of those I love engirth me and I engirth them,
They will not let me off till I go with them, respond to them,
And discorrupt them, and charge them full with the charge
of the soul.

So wrote Walt Whitman nearly 120 years ago.

Denie Hiestand is the most compelling, stimulating, frustrating, exhilarating, exasperating author I've read since D. H. Lawrence. It seems, based upon the many accounts I've read, that he's the same in person as was Lawrence. Agree or disagree with his methods and conclusions — or better still, find yourself engaged in a continuing dialogue with his words — and you'll be better off for the experience. Just be ready for a wild ride.

Unlike his conclusions, Denie's journey is irrefutable. The voyage took place. And his message, at first glance so radical, is actually deeply conservative, going back to the Atomists of Plato's era, Jesus and the Fathers of Christianity, and the core writings of Hinduism and Zen. It embraces the physics of Einstein and the quantum mechanics of Feynman, which Einstein couldn't do.

His message is so simple, it takes two books, so far, to help the reader scrape away centuries of rationalistic encrustation to convey it. The universe is energy. We are part of the universe. We are energy. Connect truthfully with the energy that is *both* you and the so-called "universe," and you can finally live a healthy, unfragmented life.

Sound too easy, too simple? Recall the words of a great philosopher, Lao Tzu: "The way that can be sought is not the Way." Read *Journey to Truth* so you can understand how hard-won his insights are. Read *Electrical Nutrition* to learn how to apply them to improving your health. Suspend your disbelief until what he says has time to sink in. Then, while you may feel like arguing this point or that, arguments he'd surely relish, just *try* to disbelieve that this man had made the journey he describes and by which he lives.

— ROBERT KALAN, MA.ED.,
author of *Jump, Frog, Jump; Rain;* and *Blue Sea*

Preface

To many people, the concept of nutrition being an electrical process may be difficult to grasp. It was not so long ago that I was part of that group. Perhaps the best way to explain vibrational medicine is to give you a brief outline of how I learned about our electrical make-up.

I was introduced to vibrational medicine, the umbrella term for all the healing techniques pertaining to the electrical function of the body, when some years ago I suffered severe depression combined with an almost total shutdown of my physical systems, resulting in very real self-destructive tendencies. A common term used to describe this multisystem "disease" is *chronic fatigue syndrome*.

The result of my going to hell and back was that I was left with a deep inner drive that compelled me to study and learn to understand what causes the body to stop working, the emotions to go out of control, and "disease" to set in. I was gently and lovingly made aware that humans have the ability (sometimes with a little help) to heal and function as complete beings on a physical, emotional, and spiritual level.

I have been on an incredible journey of self-awareness, understanding, and knowledge that in turn has made me realize that what has helped me can help others and that I can use my knowledge to assist others on their own path of healing. I enrolled in specialized courses in yoga; massage; cell electrology (the study of the cells' energy systems); Shen physio-emotional release therapy; awareness release therapy; color, herb, crystal, and naturopathic therapies; cell function physiology; lymphology; electrical stress release; and other energy healing methods. I also read everything I could get my hands on and studied many other health and healing techniques. As a result of years of study, I became qualified to practice a type of homeopathy called homeobotanical therapy, became a certified cell electrology instructor, and obtained a certificate of lymphology. Continuing my studies and always looking to expand my horizons, I went on to gain more experience and qualifications in energy mastery and vibrational medicine, including training with Robert Jaffe, M.D., founder of the Jaffe Institute of Spiritual and Medical Healing, and practical implementation with over 15,000 clients worldwide.

It was soon obvious to me that all of these therapies that I was studying were utilizing life-force energy in one form or another in its various frequencies, often without the therapist realizing or understanding that this energy was being used.

Before this, I had spent a lifetime in the farming industry keeping animals healthy. I owned and operated at different times several very successful farms with 500 dairy cows, 2,500 deer, and 3,000 sheep, along with an agricultural contracting business.

As humans are indeed a type of animal, I soon realized that many of the concepts that I utilized in keeping my animals healthy could be directly applied to the human health-care field. I have implemented these insights, along with the understanding that we are electrical and that this is an electrical universe, in my health practice over the years. I now have over 15,000 people in my client base who have put these principles into practice and who have benefited from them dramatically. These ideas are direct from nature, and they work, as nature in all her glory works. Electrical nutrition is a key component in the electrical reconstruction of the body, and this concept will be discussed in depth throughout this book.

Because of the processes I have been through and the burning vision within my heart, I know that our inheritance is health in all its wonderful, glorious, joyful manifestations. Perfect health and vitality is our natural state of being.

Then why is it that record numbers of people are dying of cancer and other degenerative diseases? Why is it that people in the Western world are spending more on health-related problems now than in any other time in history? Why is disease in all its manifestations at an all-time high? Why is it that Western society is riddled with discontent, emotional dis-empowerment (feeling emotionally weak and victimized), and, for most, financial enslavement? Why is it that the human experience has left most of the people on this earth, particularly those living in the Western hemisphere, with a sense of abandonment and disconnection from self and in a state of despair? How is it that the greatest industrial achievements this earth has seen have left our world disharmonious, polluted, toxic, and out of step with every aspect of nature? Is this truly what we would call civilization? Is this truly the way we want to live life? Is this in any way "getting it right"? I suggest that it is not.

In this book I share with you my explanations for why we are in this unholy mess and why it is that everywhere I look, I see human beings struggling with their very existence. I share with you what I perceive to be erroneous concepts within our so-called sciences and my ideas about how these false perceptions came to be.

I hope you will be able to see a different reality, an electrical reality, a way out of the mire, a way back to life, by following your journey to truth and embracing electrical nutrition.

—DENIE HIESTAND, founder,
International Institute of Vibrational Wellness

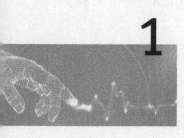

1

Electrical Nutrition and Vibrational Medicine

Our life-force energy is a subtle form of electromagnetic energy. It is the animating current of life without which we do not exist. This energy is not a recent discovery. Through the centuries, it has been called different names by many people: Christ called it "light." The Russians in their psychic research have called it bioplasmic energy. Austrian psychoanalyst Wilhelm Reich referred to it as orgone energy. East Indian yogis call it *prana*. The Chinese call it *chi*. Ancient alchemists spoke of the "vital fluid," and Bruner (a well-known German scientist) named it "biocosmic energy." Hippocrates called it "nature's life-force." Antoine Bechamp, who may be considered the father of our modern drug-based medical system, recognized it as all of life, the key that all else revolved around. I am sure there are many other names for this energy, but for the purposes of this book, I call it vibrational energy, or our electrical life force.

1

This life-force energy flows through the body as if it were following an invisible wiring system, charging every cell in its path. This electrical system is referred to as meridians as it pulses through the body, and the aura, an electromagnetic energy field, that surrounds the body. This electrical current can become weakened or partially blocked. When this happens, illness, physical malfunction, pain, and emotional problems develop. Vibrational medicine does not focus on the symptoms but rather focuses directly on the energy/electrical system to restore and reconstruct the correct electrical flow.

UNDERSTANDING VIBRATIONAL MEDICINE

Vibrational medicine, also called energy medicine, is the use of several therapeutic modalities to determine where and why the body's energy flow is disturbed and to reestablish the proper flow and alignment of the life force throughout the body. It is all about moving away from limitations, labels, and boxes in health care and toward embracing all of what we are and all of what is known. It is about how we can care for, repair, and assist each other to function fully as empowered and healthy individuals.

I believe that advanced electrical knowledge of the body and how to repair the electrical malfunctions—which is, in fact, what all disease, pain, and physical problems are but symptoms of—is the biggest, most important requirement in any health-care learning process that one can now undertake. The cells in the body work electrically, not chemically. Therefore, pain, impaired movement, illness, or disease—as we tend to label these malfunctions—are the result of low electrical energy in the cells. Pain in all its manifestations is real, but often a physical reason for it is not apparent. This is perfectly understandable when we realize that our bodies are electrical and that our experience of physicality is only our limited perception of this reality.

Everything is energy, and all energy has the ability to communicate. Practicing vibrational medicine is simply a matter of becoming aware of the natural energy communications occurring at all times. It is about being able to develop one's natural ability to read the energy of the human body and focus and direct and be receptive to very subtle frequencies that are part of our universe.

Science tells us that energy follows awareness (that is how mind power works). This theory, combined with an understanding of the workings of the physical body, helps vibrational medicine practitioners understand the electrical workings of the cells and the energy function of the atom at the subcellular level. With this knowledge, it is possible to become aware of the electrical energy within the cell. Once this connection is made, since energy follows awareness, as long as awareness is held and the energy connection is maintained, energy can be focused into any cell or group of cells.

The natural healing arts, or complementary medicine, are becoming increasingly combined under the heading of *vibrational medicine*, and all the different modalities are but pieces of the puzzle that make up the big picture. The big picture is how the body works at its most real and deepest level, the subatomic electrical level, and its reconstruction at this core level is vibrational medicine.

TRACING THE ORIGINAL ELECTRICAL CAUSE OF ILLNESS

The electrical cause of disease states has always been of special interest to me. (I am often referred to as the "body electrician.") Drawing on my experience of working with the body's electromagnetic energy system, I am able to follow the energy matrix of the disease backward to the original trauma. In many cases, the electrical problem started years ago. It took that long for enough cells to be electrically damaged and for enough circuits to "blow their fuses" before the problem manifested as the physical disease. There is not a disease state that is not evident in the body's electromagnetic energy fields prior to its physical manifestation. A human being is an electrical apparatus. The frequency we vibrate at gives us our physicality.

Electromagnetic frequencies of the body's system can be measured by those specialized in that field with extremely sensitive scientific equipment, or one can be taught how to become aware of vibrating frequencies of energy. Tuning in to the energy of another human being is very much a learned art for those who are prepared to put in the time and effort. Once one has mastered this ability, the root cause of disease manifestations becomes much easier to ascertain.

Our present medical model has absolutely no way of figuring out the chain of events that lead to the physical manifestation of a problem. A trained vibrational medicine practitioner is able to access the information contained within the energy fields of the body. Through this communication, it is possible to follow the frequencies back in order to learn when and how the original trauma took place.

My ability to trace disease symptoms back to their original electrical malfunctions has enabled me to see certain patterns. Many of our common disease states can be dramatically alleviated by understanding some of these basic patterns, which express the fundamentals of the way nature works.

VIBRANT HEALTH—OUR BIRTHRIGHT

We all seek good health—the fullest expression of the life force that is available to us. Anything less than this is a state of dis-ease. Now look around you. Can you honestly say that there are many people who exhibit this full expression of life? Do you know any people who exude life from every pore of their being? Who are so vibrant and full of energy that they charge the atmosphere of a room when they walk in, or simply make you feel better by being around them? Maybe there are a handful of these healthy, happy souls, but it certainly is not the norm.

This state of vibrant health is our birthright. At our core level, we are vibrant, alive, positive, and happy. But, sadly, life's experiences and the stress of daily existence cause our bodies to degenerate, our emotions to go AWOL, and our souls to feel disconnected.

All too often, this is a reality in today's society. But with the information in this book, you will be able to make life-affirmative choices, start to rebuild your physicality, and reverse the degenerative process. Once again, life can become pleasurable.

MEDICAL MYTHS AND MISCONCEPTIONS

First, I am going to ask you to look at some of the modern health myths and question the modern concepts of how our bodies work; to take what we know and perhaps turn it inside out; to look at things from another angle and to stretch the parameters of your very thought processes and beliefs. Why? Because after all the time that humans have walked this earth, our current state of disease and degeneration suggest that it is time we summon up the courage to challenge the premises on which we have based those beliefs.

A Particle Universe? . . .

One premise that common science is based on, that of a "particle universe," may be erroneous. In the particle universe mentality, everything is separate, isolated, and disconnected. Cause and full effect are often not taken into consideration, as when a drug is given to address one problem in the body but produces side effects in other parts. Or when we discard toxic waste into the ocean, and the fish subsequently develop heavy-metal toxicity, which affects those who eat them. People often do not associate environmental pollution with resulting disease. Another example could be that of a hand cream containing petroleum jelly. Initially, nobody realized that the benzene, which gets absorbed through the skin, would subsequently be found to be a carcinogen (a cancer-causing agent). The hand cream may have worked very well, but there was another cause and effect in operation that was not immediately apparent.

An objective look at basic chemistry would suggest that this is not a particle universe—when two components are combined, the resulting combination can look and react in a way that neither of the original parts would have suggested. For example, if we take two molecules of hydrogen, which is an explosive gas, and one molecule of oxygen, which is the gas required for combustion (burning), you would think that adding them together would make a very big bang or a big fire. In theory, this would seem to be the case—in practice, however, we see that quite the opposite happens. When we combine them, we make water (H_2O). The combination creates a very different physical reality than the sum of the individual components. Water is neither explosive nor helpful in the burning process. The combination reacts and creates something entirely different.

. . . An Electrical Universe!

The above example would suggest that we need to look further into what is actually taking place. How did this seemingly impossible change take place? To help us do this, first let's look at what the body is made of. We were all taught that the body is made of cells, and that cells are made of atoms. So far so good, but what are atoms made of? Atoms are made up of electrical impulses spinning around each other called protons, electrons, and neutrons. Groups of atoms are called molecules. The way these protons, neutrons, and electrons are arranged or configured is called the electrical matrix; and the speed at which they spin around each other could be loosely termed their vibratory rate or frequency.

When a reconfiguration or change in the electrical matrix takes place, as in when two groups of molecules are combined (two hydrogen and one oxygen molecule) the frequency and the resulting physicality also changes. What we perceive as different things is really only a different configuration of the electrical matrix of the atomic structure. Every part of every cell that makes up our body, and in fact every part of everything in the known universe, is made up of these electrical impulses. This is an electrical universe.

In a particle universe mindset, we think that one and one makes two; but in an "electrical universe," we would say that one and one has made "one." As in the water example above, two components, the hydrogen and the oxygen, have combined to create something that is now completely different from the original individual components. This new combination does not look or behave in any way that resembles the individual parts, but is rather a brand new and different *singular* whole.

This electrical understanding is not necessarily applied to drugs or their use in mainstream medicine. Quite often, individual ingredients that on their own produce certain effects in the body, when combined and taken internally have a completely different effect from what was originally envisioned. Many times, mainstream medications are ineffective or produce a toxic effect due to their incompatible electrical configurations. This electrical understanding is only now being incorporated into the formulation of some herbal and nutritional supplements so that the combinations of different herbs are compatible electrically with the body and create the desired results. This has been achieved by a handful of scientists who are aware of this electrical reality and have conducted a lifetime of research on combining different herbs and natural ingredients. This electrical formulating concept, which is now available to the public, is at the forefront of natural health research. See Appendix A for information on companies from whom you can obtain such products.

It was 2,700 years ago that Thales, the great Greek philosopher, started to philosophize about what the universe was made of. Science today is still based on his premise that this is an isolated particle universe. Yet in reality, there are no separate particles in the entire cosmos—everything is interrelated and connected. Every thing—*everything*—is made of atoms, and atoms are made of *vibrating frequencies of energy* (electrical impulses). Energy is everything, and everything is energy.

Every frequency (speed of vibration) of energy interfaces with, is affected by, and is connected seamlessly to every other frequency of energy. This is an electrical universe. There is not, there never was, there never will be, and there cannot be an individual thing that is unrelated to anything in this cosmos. There is no separation. All energy is a part of all other energy.

Have we been going down the wrong path with the wrong concepts? If the universe is made of energy, then surely we must question current science and its hypotheses. If modern medicine, food production, and manufacturing are based on incorrect science, then is it any wonder that we are experiencing ever greater levels of degeneration and disease?

The only way we can truly understand our world, our universe, and ourselves is to understand it from an energy perspective. The only way we can ever hope to truly understand our bodies is from an energy perspective. The only way we can ever alleviate disease is to approach it from an energy perspective. The only way to formulate our supplements and our medicine is to approach it from an energy perspective. The only way we can make this world into the Garden of Eden is to view it from an energy perspective.

By helping you see that there is another concept, another logic that we can embrace, I hope to help you gain the ability to move beyond the boxes of our limited belief structures. If we can understand that we are electrical, that this is an electrical universe, and that everything we do is electrically/energetically based, then everything about our lives — our health and the way we think, feel, process, and live as human beings — has the potential to change. To change the concepts that make up our logic, to change the premise our consciousness is based on, is to change consciousness itself, and with that our world.

When we become aware of this new premise, that of an electrical universe, and adopt this new consciousness, we begin to realize just who we are and what we are made of. Life can be disease and pain free. Life truly can be an experience that we, products of this electrical universe, have a right to live with total joy.

"Traditional" Medicine, Another Modern Myth

Having dispatched the concept of the particle universe, we can move onto another of the modern myths — "traditional medicine." In Western society, the term *traditional medicine* is often used to describe our drug-based medical care system. However, tradition is defined as a belief, a principle, or a way of acting that people in a particular society or group have followed for a long time.

To call our present medical system a "traditional" system is, I believe, a misrepresentation. Our present medical system has only been with us since the early 1900s. Medical drugs and their use have only come to dominate our health care in the last fifty years. Our modern drug-based medical system is not based on any long-term history or ancient knowledge. Many of the medical drugs that were used in this country thirty years ago are no longer used because of their discovered toxic effects.

Our modern drug-based system is the newest, most untried, most unproven, most untraditional health-care system in the world. It could be considered one of the most dangerous experiments ever conducted on an unsuspecting populace.

There is nothing traditional, nothing ancient, nothing steeped in antiquity about any part of our modern health care. It uses incredibly powerful and toxic substances that the body has no ability to recognize as nutrition, with absolutely no thought given to the electrical bombardment the body suffers as a result of digesting, being injected with, or being exposed to these concoctions.

MODERN MEDICINES ARE
ELECTRICAL HAND GRENADES

The chemical compounds that make up our modern medicines hold within them such powerful active ingredients that the body often responds as if an electrical hand grenade had been detonated within. This electrical damage manifests as many different physical symptoms, which are medically labeled "side effects." Often, these side effects are as devastating, or more so, than the original problem. Sadly, they sometimes become apparent only years later.

When prescribing drugs for us, our medical practitioners often do not adequately inform us of the dangers and possible toxic effects of them. I have had to deal with major manifestations of these problems—as serious as liver and kidney damage and potential failure—many times in my clinical experience. One example springs to mind of a reasonably healthy male, who, under a relatively high degree of stress, developed heartburn symptoms. He had been prescribed a drug that, unbeknownst to him, had the side effect of causing severe stomach ulceration if taken over a long period.

After three years on this drug, this reasonably healthy man developed severe stomach pain and was eventually diagnosed as having chronic stomach ulcers. The destruction to his stomach was so severe that a succession of five operations resulted in the removal of two-thirds of his stomach and intestinal tract. The resulting lack of digestive ability led to toxic effects throughout his body, and he was prescribed more and more drugs to suppress the increasing number of side effects that developed. This eventually led to kidney and liver damage, which became life threatening. His wife, who researched the available medical literature, later learned that severe stomach ulceration was a side effect of the originally prescribed drug if taken for a period longer than *four to six weeks*.

Sadly, it is often only when death is a very real possibility that people search for alternate options. This man was basically knocking on death's door by the time he found his way to my clinic. Generally, rebuilding the electrical function of organs such as the liver and kidneys is usually not too difficult; however, the removal of the toxic residue and the rebuilding of the cells damaged by this drug concoction that had been prescribed over many years was a slow and difficult process.

We were able to help this man to become relatively drug free and to regain some semblance of a life. However, because of the severity of the drug-induced damage to a large part of his system, he was never a healthy man again and, after much battling, he finally succumbed to liver and kidney failure. The surviving family now holds traditional medicine in contempt.

It should be understood that I am not out to bash modern medicine, nor am I *totally* against it. Thanks to modern medicine, we have an incredible amount of information about the workings of the body and specific disorders that was unavailable to us before. The knowledge in organ transplant technology and traumatic accident care is without a doubt extremely advantageous and helpful to many people. There are also many thousands of doctors who conscientiously work very diligently not to overprescribe and abuse the power they have in administering powerful, and in some cases toxic, drugs.

It would be a wonderful world if all the knowledge from all the known health-care systems and modalities were an accepted part of one overall health-care system. I fail to see why there is a need for division and antagonistic attitudes between the different modalities. Is not the goal to assist people back to a state of good health? Surely the only honest way that assistance can be given is by sharing the benefits of the knowledge that all of humanity has amassed.

MEDICAL MISADVENTURES

A good 50 percent of the clients I have seen in my clinics in the last fifteen years have come to me as a result of medically induced problems. When all else fails, our present medical system cuts out the malfunctioning part and throws it away, suggesting that nature got it wrong and we really did not need that part in the first place. Looking at the medical misadventures abounding and the misinformation we are all fed, it is easy to understand that our present medical model possibly is based on some incorrect foundations.

During the ten-year period of the Vietnam War, approximately 5,000 Americans lost their lives per year. Up to 360,000 Americans die *every year* as a result of medical misadventure in American hospitals. These people did not die as a result of the problems they were originally admitted into the hospital for but of other medical- and drug-induced mistakes and problems. There was an outcry over the 5,000 casualties per year in Vietnam, yet I am astounded by the lack of voices protesting the devastation of the general populace by the present medical system.

A report published by the *Journal of American Medical Association* (*JAMA*) affirmed that an estimated 2,216,000 hospital patients experienced a serious adverse drug reaction (ADR) each year.[1] The authors defined a serious ADR as one that requires hospitalization, prolongs hospitalization, is permanently disabling, or results in death. Furthermore, they estimate that ADRs cause a minimum of more than 106,000 deaths in the United States alone, making ADRs between the fourth and sixth greatest cause of death in the United States. And they call it medicine!

Another report, in the *Archives of Internal Medicine*, pointed out that preventable illness and death from the misuse of medicines cost the American economy over $75 billion a year.[2] If lost productivity is taken into account, the cost rises to $182 billion. The researchers point out that the purpose of prescribing pharmaceutical drugs is to treat disease successfully—not to cause more problems. They estimate that this purpose is achieved in less than 40 percent of all cases. More than 60 percent of all people prescribed pharmaceutical drugs end up with a drug-related problem, which results in almost nine million hospital admissions a year. As a matter of fact, more that 28 percent of all hospital admissions in 1992 were due to drug-related illness, and somewhere between 80,000 and 200,000 people died from doctor-prescribed medicines. The researchers conclude that drug-related illness and death should be considered one of the leading "diseases" in the United States.

SELECTIVE EDUCATION

The pharmaceutical industry has become so powerful that the knowledge of the electrical workings of the body and other natural health practices is largely unavailable in our "traditional" medical training institutions. Thousands of years of knowledge in the field of herbal medicine have been denied to us by the same medical control mechanisms. Even the nutritional understanding known in veterinary medicine twenty years ago is still not taught in our medical schools. Nutrition is the basis of life. Yet our medical professionals, who are legislated by law to be the guardians of our vitality, have had little knowledge (four hours on nutrition out of seven years' medical training) to provide us so that we could promote that very vitality.

The knowledge of the electrical workings of our bodies has been taken by some sectors of our modern scientific community to heights never before discovered, yet not one part of this electrical knowledge pertaining to the human body is taught in any of the "traditional" medical learning institutions in North America.

The knowledge of vibrational medicine has been perfected over thousands of years by many cultures. The Chinese for many centuries have had an understanding of the electrical functions of the body and have used this understanding as a basis for a holistic approach to health care in acupuncture. The healing properties of botanicals, essential oils, the laying on of hands, and minerals and vitamins have, by and large, been excluded from our current medical paradigm by the enactment of laws. Yet the most dangerous, life-twisting drugs are injected and ingested with the full backing of the very same laws.

The move to severely restrict the availability of herbs and other natural health products or services should be thwarted. Any such arbitrary limitations we allow to permeate our lives and our society becomes a limitation of our own life force, which in turn affects each and every cell in our bodies. The restriction of life force to our cells impacts our electrical circuitry with the effect of reducing the flow of energy throughout the body and thus promotes disease.

One of the most basic and oldest forms of nurturing is the beautiful art of massage. The touching of one human by another has a profound and measurable effect on all connective tissue, and assists the flow of oxygen, lymph fluid, and health. In many of the states in the United States, very restrictive laws limit and control—and indeed criminalize—citizens who are not "licensed" to use this most natural and beautiful healing art. Surely there is something amiss when society allows legal control to be placed on the honorable touch between two consenting human beings.

SUMMARY

We are electrical, and this is an electrical universe, in which everything is interconnected. Disease states are nothing more than an electrical malfunction, and vibrational medicine addresses the causes of these malfunctions, not just the symptoms. Modern medicines can have the effect of an electrical hand grenade in the body, whereas electrical nutrition will help bring the body back into harmony. We have been fed many health care mistruths and have accepted a health-care system that seems to have promoted more disharmony, toxic effects, and death in the human body than ever before. Many of the malfunctions that occur in the body are due to incorrect fermentation. We will now discuss the electrical process of digestion so that you can start to take responsibility, take back your power, and regain your health and vitality.

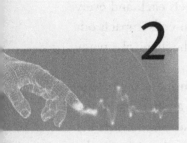

2

Nourishment—An Electrical Process

Digestion could be considered *the* most important function in the body, since compromised digestion affects the health of the entire body. The process commonly referred to as digestion is actually fermentation of the eaten food. The term *fermentation* scientifically refers to a very basic process of breaking food down into its constituent elements—rotting, if you will. In essence, the function of our digestive tract is to control the "rotting" of the food we eat.

In this chapter, first, we will look at the evolution of different food sources and their available life force relative to their rotting ability. Then we will address the electrical process of digestion and how the food transfers its energy to us.

What follows is probably a very new way of thinking for most people and perhaps is difficult to "digest." However, the laws of quantum physics, even, would support these concepts. We will try to explain these seemingly difficult energy concepts as simply as possible.

THE ROCK-TO-ROT THEORY

A great Chinese philosopher has been quoted as saying, "First I was a rock, then I was a plant, then I was an animal, and now I am me." Perhaps this little phrase contains the truth of our very existence.

If everything is energy, and all energy interfaces with all other energy, this means our body has evolved within the electrical reality pertaining to this earth. If you like, it had to evolve as part of what we would call nature.

When we look at our nutritional base and follow the chain of nutritional availability backward, we find that every form of nutrition on this planet originated as inorganic matter. Or, put simply, food on this planet started out as a rock. All our nutrition comes from this source.

Like everything in existence, a rock also consists of vibrating frequencies of energy, so in that sense it is alive. However, the frequency of a rock is such that its constituent nutritional components are vibrating so slowly, they are unavailable to us directly. From an electrical nutrition point of view, the nutritional availability of food is indexed to its vibratory rate (frequency).

Everything consists of atoms, which are vibrating frequencies of energy, however the frequency varies from one form of existence to another, so perhaps it is possible to look at the life force of everything on earth in terms of its frequency. At one end of this scale we have very low frequency forms of life called rocks, and at the opposite end of this scale we have humans, the highest frequency life form. Looking at this evolution from a nutritional point of view, every life form between these two extremes has an important and naturally structured place in the increasing vibratory rate scale, from the inorganic rock to the flesh and bones that make up our bodies.

Looking at it another way, the lowest form of life on this planet is that which does not rot—a rock. That which is the most evolved away from the rock, with the highest vibratory rate, is that which decays the most rapidly, such as flesh. For example, if we place on the ground outside a rock, some wheat and other grains, some vegetables, some fruit, and some animal flesh—which do you think would rot (decay) the quickest? The rock would still be there in a million years; the grains would be there for months, if not years; some of the vegetables would not rot for days or even weeks (some would last longer, like carrots and potatoes); the fruit would go bad in days. At the other end of the scale, the flesh would decay in a matter of hours. From an electrical nutrition standpoint, the quicker the food rots, the more evolved it is, the higher the vibration rate it contains, and the greater the life force it has available to us.

Rocks, which consist of inorganic compounds, have in them every known mineral needed for our nourishment. However, because of the rock's low frequency, its compounds and minerals are unavailable to us. We would die eating rocks.

It could be said that the food chain is started by the lichen and other fungi that gnaw into and live on the rocks. The lichen and fungi refine the nutrients of the rock and the nutrients then become incorporated into their life.

Then come the plants that take up the nutrients left behind by the decaying lichen and fungi. The plants evolve this food one more step, increasing its vibratory rate one more notch. Thus this food becomes part of the plant's body. Plants, from an energy understanding, are higher in vibratory rate (more evolved) than rocks.

Then along comes the animal, which eats the plant and refines its constituent products even further. The vibratory rate of the plant increases even more and is now bounding around as an animal. Animal flesh, as pointed out earlier, decays much faster than does plant life.

We now have a demonstration that shows us that as life evolves away from the rock, it becomes less like it. As the frequency increases, its vibratory rate can be indexed to an increase in rotting ability, which demonstrates its movement away from the frequency of the rock. This is natural evolution.

We then come along and eat the animals and take that evolutionary stage one step further. The animal then becomes part of our life, which could be considered the highest vibratory rate life form on this planet—we are at the top of the food chain.

THE ELECTRICAL REALITY OF FOOD

From a nutritional point of view, everything we do to our food changes its subtle electrical reality, its electrical matrix, its frequency, its energy (power) and how it interfaces with our body. The way we fertilize it, spray it, drench it, heat it, wash it, dry it, mix it, take bits out of it, put bits into it, irradiate it, preserve it, color it, flavor it, freeze it, etc., changes the food's electrical matrix. Even what we store food in and every human contact the food has affects its electrical makeup. From the farmer who touched the seed or the animal, to the check-out person at the supermarket, all have infused a frequency of energy into that food. Then, of course, the person who is preparing the food for our ingestion has a profound effect on its frequency, as well (the movie *Like Water for Chocolate* is a wonderful depiction of this).

Let's look at water as an example of what happens when a substance's electrical matrix is changed. If we look at ice, water, and vapor, we can see that as we change the electrical matrix (or the frequency) of a water molecule, the resulting physicality and its interface with everything around it changes. If you do not think ice has a different physicality from water, I am sure that if he was alive, the captain of the Titanic would give you a good argument.

We can breathe water molecules as in humidity, but we cannot see it. Water in its liquid state, however, would kill us if we tried to breathe it, yet we cannot survive without drinking it. And ice (water in solid form) would break our bones if we tried diving in it, and I have never seen a fish swim in ice.

In another example, if we melt tin, which melts at 449° F, and lead, which has a melting point of 621° F, and then mix the two molten materials together and allow them to solidify, the resulting alloy (solder) will be very different from the two components we started with.

The behavior, or physical properties, of our new alloy, solder, is exceedingly different from either of the two components, or their sum total. In other words, everything about it now is different. The most startling physical difference is solder's melting point, which is 361° F— way below that of tin or lead. The resulting solder is also a much softer metal than either of its original components. What has actually changed is its electrical matrix—the way its neutrons, protons, and electrons are arranged and thus behave.

So you see, as soon as we change the frequency of anything, we change the way it then interfaces with everything else. In other words, to change the electrical construct of protons and electrons, is to change everything about them—their physicality, appearance, and what we perceive them to be.

Nature, which we are a part of, designed an electrical synergy between the food chain and ourselves that allows the energy that is the nutritional frequencies of the food to be seamlessly available to us. Our so-called technology, particularly in the last thirty years, has dramatically changed the electrical matrix of every piece of food we buy from the supermarket, resulting in our bodies decreased ability to recognize it as perfect energy-giving food.

Hopefully, it is becoming glaringly obvious that we are unconsciously poisoning ourselves. Due to the fact that our education system focuses primarily on physics and chemistry, the electrical understanding of what food is and what it does has not been taken into consideration. When we look at every aspect of our present environment, we have to come to the conclusion that we have changed everything we interface with. As you understand more about electrical nutrition, you will gain the knowledge that will enable you to make positive choices of which foods are electrically available.

THE WAY IT WAS

Two hundred years ago, before the advent of modern agriculture, everything we planted, grew, and ate contained the electrical matrix nature had developed over tens of thousands of years. All of our medicine came from the knowledge of herbs that had been built up since time began. There was hardly any evidence of many of the diseases and problems we live with today, such as cancer, fibromyalgia, cystic fibrosis, PMS, AIDS, multiple sclerosis, autism, Alzheimer's disease, and many of the other degenerative disorders that plague modern society.

The water consumed back then was completely free of the toxins from our modern industrial age that have absolutely no electrical synergy with the body, including chlorine, acetone, chloride, carbon tetrachloride, mercury, lead, aluminum, fluoride, and petrochemical distillates.

When the pioneer farmers first started to plow the Midwest plains in the United States, there was more than six feet of topsoil. Today there is much less and its mineral base is gone. The fruits and vegetables that are commercially grown in North America (and most of the world) do not have the same genetic makeup, or contain the same electrical matrix that nourished our great-grandparents.

A good starting point to correct this electrical and dietary disharmony would be to supplement with electrically available minerals, herbs, enzymes, and natural bacteria.

THE "ELECTRICS" OF DIGESTION

To understand digestion from an electrical perspective, it is important to recall that every cell, every molecule, and every atom consists of energy. These energy impulses are arranged (their electrical matrix) in a way that enables us to see it as physical. This physicality that we are aware of, is only a very small part of the total energy that makes up everything—including our food. Every atom that makes up each food particle has its own unique frequency. It is this energy that is transferred to us and is our nourishment.

Physical food never ever gets anywhere near our cells. The large majority of what we perceive as food (its physical aspect) passes out through our bowels as physical waste. The digestion process allows the food particles (molecules—little bundles of vibrating energy) to begin their journey to become our life.

To understand the importance of fermentation, we need to look at the process in some depth. The digestive process starts in the mouth. Humans, not unlike cows, have flat, grinding teeth and jaws that can move sideways, allowing grinding motion. Only the animals with a digestive tract capable of fermenting vegetation have this grinding ability. This is because the only part of the vegetation that is available to nourish us is an incredibly small molecule inside the cell.

To extract this single molecule (with its energy field intact), we first have to grind the vegetation with our teeth to break open the outside wall of the cell. Then when we swallow, the partially ground matter gets combined with the live enzymes and digestive bacteria, as well as the gastric juices, which then complete the fermentation process, allowing the release of the small molecule from within the cell. As the molecule is released from the cell, its energy field is electrically attracted (like iron filings to a magnet) to the field of energy surrounding the cells of the stomach and intestinal lining. It is then electrically drawn to and passes through the microscopic pores of the linings, from there passing into the bloodstream. The remaining fiber is then disposed of through our bowels.

THE ELECTRICAL SPARK

The little molecule is now being pumped around our blood system and eventually goes down one of the millions of side roads called capillaries that lead to every cell. Capillaries are very porous. Their holes are small enough, however, to prevent most of the blood components, such as water (the biggest constituent) and the red and white blood cells, from passing through. But most of our food molecules do pass through—into the lymphatic fluid that surrounds all of our cells.

At this point something truly amazing happens—something that is rarely addressed by mainstream science or nutritionists. The little molecule now absorbs solar energy and in fact acts just like a capacitor in the ignition system of some vehicles. It builds up within itself a charge of energy that has the potential to be exponentially far greater than its original charge (much like sound impulses from a microphone going through an amplifier and coming out much louder). However, it still carries within its electrical matrix the original frequency of the food it started out as. In some ways, this is not electrically dissimilar to the process of photosynthesis occurring in plants. When we are denied solar energy, as miners are when working underground at a depth of 500 feet or more, many degenerative diseases rapidly manifest, regardless of perceived adequate nutrition. This is why mining laws are still in place to limit the hours that deep mine workers may spend underground.

If the food was properly fermented, its surrounding energy field will have a positive charge. The field surrounding a healthy cell has a negative charge. As we move, our lymphatic fluid is pumped throughout the body, moving the molecule around and causing it to brush past a cell. What happens next is the same as lightning. Since the fields of energy surrounding the molecule and the cell are oppositely charged, the molecule zaps out a spark of energy into the cell, and the cell zaps back its spark. At this point, the molecule's field of energy should undergo a polarity reversal (meaning its field of energy is now negatively charged).

This process is similar to a spark plug in your car's gasoline engine, where energy (the spark) jumps from one polarity to another (a positively charged component to a negatively charged component). Without it the engine would not be able to function, the fuel would not become motive power for the car, and in your body you would not get the life force from the food.

In traditional science, this spark reaction is called the sodium/potassium pump, referring to the process by which the cells take in the nourishment and export the waste product. However, sodium does not actually enter the cells, nor does potassium come out of the cells in physical form. It is the energy of the elements that is transferred. As matter is condensed energy, science perceives that condensation as the physical elements.

This process is an incredibly involved energy transfer. The frequency of the original food carried within the energy field of the molecule has now been discharged into the cell. It interacts with our subtle unseen energy, reconfigures, and becomes our life force. If you like, all of the constituent products that were required by the body from the food have now been transferred electrically to the body. The process is 100-percent electrical. It is not a chemical reaction.

Particle physics has no way of explaining this complex electrical process. From an electrical point of view, an entire consciousness undertakes a change, in other words, the food molecule (energy impulse) transforms into the life force of a human being. This is the only way we get fully nourished. This is the true dance of creation, an incredibly complex and instantaneous life-producing electrical transfer. Science has a very limited understanding of this, and to view the process as strictly a physical process is an oversimplification.

This is the crux of electrical nutrition and the electrical understanding of life. This is where we will be able to see and learn the properties of life and disease manifestation in the future. I believe this is twenty-first-century science in the making.

Nobel prize winners for medicine, Dr. Erwin Neher and Dr. Burt Sackmann, cell physiologists from Germany, revolutionized modern biology by contributing to the understanding of the cellular mechanisms underlying diseases. These researchers demonstrated that cells actually communicate with each other and in fact use a very complex communication system that utilizes impulses (vibrating frequencies of energy), and these impulses contain within them their own consciousness and intelligence. Also, in his book *The Body Electric: Electromagnetism and the Foundation of Life*, author and researcher Robert O. Becker, M.D., presented his lifetime of scientific research into the electrical and energetic reality of all cell function.

Therefore, the leading scientists of the world are moving away from the biological/chemical understanding of life and are heading in the direction of electrical science and electrical nutrition. Maybe science is catching up with what I am able to see electrically (energetically) in the body. I recognize that the electrical functioning of the body is very difficult to explain in a language that is based on biology and chemistry; however the biological/chemical language is the only language we have available to us to express these concepts. From the standpoint of electrical nutrition, there is no physical, biological, or chemical reaction in any part of our physicality—there is only electrical action. The physical, biological, and chemical reaction as we perceive it to be, is only the third dimensional way of perceiving, quantifying, and attempting to understand an incredibly complex and hereto largely unknown electrical universe.

It is an electrical attraction, an electrical interface, an electrical communication that is taking place. The whole process is so much more in-depth and complicated than general nutritional/medical science has ever contemplated. Medical science has little concept of this amazing dance of energy. It could be said that this is the magic of life, the mystery that allows one form of physicality to become another. This, surely, is nature at its best.

OPTIMAL CONDITIONS FOR ELECTRICAL DIGESTION

Our physical well-being is largely dependent on the fermentation process. As any farmer or home gardener will tell you, to correctly ferment anything, the conditions must be specific to the food being fermented. A farmer making silage from corn, which is a carbohydrate, knows that the pH required for controlled fermentation is different from that required to make silage from young grass, which is protein. Enzymes and specific bacteria are often added to regulate the pH for the different food sources to be fermented.

The body in its intrinsic intelligence knows to regulate its digestive enzymes and bacteria to control the pH balance of its digestive juices for different foods. It does this through electrical impulses sent among the cells involved. When we look at a plate of food in front of us, our senses, on the basis of our past experience, recognize whether the food is protein or carbohydrate. Even before the food gets to the mouth, the body is preparing itself for the coming ingestion. Our visual and olfactory senses, and then our taste buds and other sensory glands within our mouth cavity, send electrical messages to the digestive tract to set the correct conditions for digestion.

ELECTRICALLY UNAVAILABLE FOODS

Most of us believe that all food nourishes us. In fact, nothing could be further from the truth. Everything we eat does one of two things: it either nourishes us or poisons us. The reality is that most of the food we eat actually slowly poisons us because of overprocessing and the addition of preserving agents, which limit the degree to which the food can be digested.

Unfortunately, most of the world's vegetation (all the trees, plants, grains, and grasses) including carbohydrates, is not available to us as nutrition and is also toxic to some degree. Conversely, there are very few animals in nature whose flesh is toxic to us, although some species of fish can be. In times of old, all herbs (edible vegetation) had medicinal properties and vegetation was largely consumed for these properties, not as staples of the diet.

Foods whose natural "rotting" ability has been suppressed are not electrically available to the body. (If it cannot ferment, it cannot fire its spark.) These include foods containing sugar and other sweeteners, preservatives, stabilizers, and chemicals, plus foods that are packaged or processed, contain artificial flavoring and coloring, or in any other way have had nature's original electrical matrix altered.

THE PROBLEMS WITH COMBINING
DIFFERENT TYPES OF FOODS

As fermentation can take hours, problems arise when we take one mouthful of potatoes, bread, or pasta, which are carbohydrates, and in the next mouthful we eat meat, cheese, eggs, or tofu, which are proteins, or when we take mouthfuls of combinations of carbohydrates and proteins, as with a hamburger. These mouthfuls cannot be fermented correctly because of the protein/carbohydrate mix. When fermentation is compromised, toxins are produced because of the electrical distortion of the food particle's field of energy. This electrical distortion is the start of all degeneration and disease.

It is, therefore, easy to see that great problems arise from the typical American meat-and-potato or bread-and-meat combinations. In a physical sense, the breakdown of these foods may appear to be nutritionally normal, but when looked at from an electrical perspective, it is clear that it is not. The nucleus of the cell is physically released, but its field of energy is somewhat distorted because the enzyme, bacterial, and pH levels are not correct. The cell is not able to interact electrically with its surrounding environment as it should. This problem would be much like trying to start your car when the battery terminals are dirty. A small amount of current may flow, but chances are high that it would be slowed or distorted, and the engine would not turn over fast enough to start.

This, in effect, is what happens electrically in the gastrointestinal tract. Even though the molecule has been released from the cell of the original food, its electrical attraction to the energy surrounding the cells of the stomach lining is not strong. Therefore, its progress through to the blood is greatly inhibited or slowed down. This results in a bloated stomach among other problems.

In extreme cases, such as big holiday dinners where we inevitably overeat, the fermentation can be so compromised that electrical short circuits can occur. This can result in extremely uncomfortable feelings in the stomach. With children, the body reacts by quickly emptying its contents (vomiting). This is not so common with adults, due to the unresponsiveness of their toxic systems.

Continual overeating and eating meals that combine carbohydrates and proteins leads to the breakdown of the defenses of the cells that make up the stomach and intestinal linings. They then become physically damaged, allowing other decaying matter to seep through the porous lining of the intestinal tract into the bloodstream. This problem is sometimes referred to as leaky gut syndrome. In essence, it is due to an electrical malfunction. It can lead to low-level blood toxicity, low energy levels, hormone imbalances, acne, emotional instability, joint pain, weight gain, and many other future problems.

ELECTRICALLY DIRTY ENERGY FIELDS

As mentioned earlier, if fermentation was not carried out correctly, the food's molecule would not have been able to achieve its powerful positive charge, and the electrical matrix of the original food would not have been fully available. Its spark would have been weak. It is at this weak electrical interchange where many of our diseases and degenerative processes start.

After this weak and distorted electrical interchange, the little molecule's field of energy (around the outside of its surface) would not have changed polarity as it was meant to but would be electrically dirty (could be said to be neither positive or negative). As a result, instead of repulsing its brother and sister molecules, keeping the lymph fluid thin, the little molecule's electrical disharmony would cause it to attract and to attach itself to its neighbors, creating globules (groups of attached molecules).

This causes thick, sticky lymphatic fluid, which doesn't move very easily, causing us to feel sluggish, lethargic, and heavy. With movement, the lymphatic system will push the little molecule (from as far away as down in our little toe) through thousands of one-way valves until the molecule ends up at the subclavical valve on each side of our lower neck. The subclavical valve is the gateway through which the little molecule will pass back into the bloodstream and from there get delivered to the kidneys and then out of the body in the urine.

If the molecule did not spark correctly and its electrical field became "dirty," the kidneys could not read it as a correctly discharged food particle and would promptly send it back to the bloodstream instead of into the urinary tract. The molecule now becomes what could be called a free radical. As a result of this electrical damage, everything this free radical touches becomes electrically damaged. (Disharmony transfers its disharmony to everything it comes into contact with, as in the physical world). Consequently, the entire system comes under electrical bombardment. This is why we need to take powerful free-radical scavengers, like high dosages of electrically correct vitamin C, vitamin E, and other products that are now available (see Appendix A).

The damage to the electrical and physical function of the cells in the walls of the intestinal tract can also manifest as ulcers. The slow destruction of the electrical function of the intestinal lining and other cells often leads to the cells' inability to electrically communicate with its

DNA. The DNA contains all of the information necessary for perfect physical and electrical function. When the cells lose their ability to communicate electrically with their DNA, they, in essence, lose contact with their instruction manual, which according to vibrational medicine often leads to the eventual development of the disease we call cancer.

Downstream Effects of
Electrically Dirty Molecules

Aside from the free-radical damage that is taking place around the body, the little molecule's stickiness (mentioned earlier) and the subsequent globules that occur would be recognized as cholesterol by a doctor. The body recognizes these globules as problems within its system, and because of the stickiness brought about by the electrical disharmony, the globules attach themselves to the nice clean walls of our blood vessels (the body has to put it somewhere). It is very easy to see how blocked arteries and angina symptoms begin. Other sticky globules also end up in our joint cavities and calcify into arthritis and other joint degeneration problems. Or the kidneys, in a desperate attempt to clean up the blood, manage to hold onto some of these sticky globules, and we may end up with kidney stones.

One of the most insidious potential problems is that some of these globules get pumped around our circulatory system and, because their size is now greater than the size of the openings in the walls of the capillaries, their escape from them is impossible. The organ that has the greatest amount of these small diameter capillaries is the brain. As these globules move into the brain capillaries, they eventually get to one where the diameter is smaller than the size of the globule. This sticky mess then blocks the blood flow and the downstream tissues get starved of oxygen and nutrition. These cells can no longer function properly and can die. Initially, we call this aging. When many capillaries become blocked, you start to become concerned about your short-term memory, loss of cohesiveness, balance problems, and other "aging problems" and say your brain/body is not as good as it used to be. In extreme cases, one can have major degenerative diseases like Alzheimer's or Parkinson's disease and other motor neuron symptoms developing. All this because of incorrect fermentation, eating processed and preserved foods, and consuming carbohydrates and proteins together.

SUMMARY

When we embrace the electrical universe, we have to come to terms with the reality of everything being an electrical construct, carrying within itself an electrical matrix and interfacing with everything on an electrical or energy level. To change any component of the matrix is to effect change of the whole.

This concept totally displaces the particle physics mindset and perhaps reassigns chemistry to kindergarten logic. We live in an electrical universe, we are electrical, and everything we interface with is electrical. Everything is an electrical action, not a chemical reaction. The universe, this earth, the soil, the plants, the animals, and us, have evolved in this electrical reality we call nature. For us to be alive and healthy, the undistorted energy from all of nature has to be transferred to our bodies. Any change, any distortion, any disharmony we infuse into any part of our air, water, soil, or food is going to eventually compromise our health.

As you can see, our entire modern food-handling process, where the emphasis is on long shelf life, is in fact turning our food into poisons. All processes or inputs that limit or slow down the fermentation (rotting) of food turn food into a potential disease-causing time bomb. The alteration of the constituent ingredients of natural foods, the genetic manipulation of crops, and manufacturing and processing change the electrical function and the electrical matrix of food and make it almost impossible for our bodies to electrically recognize its energy. We are killing the spark of life that is contained in natures' bounty. Every time we allow ourselves or our children to drink a can of soda, to have a cookie, to have some candy, to eat out of a packet of preserved food, and to eat day after day a predominance of grain-based manufactured (unrottable) foods (breakfast cereal, doughnuts, pasta, bread, etc.), we are causing within our bodies electrical time bombs that will be guaranteed to slowly kill us and/or our children. Strong words, indeed, but nevertheless, sadly, deadly true!

The rapid increase in cancer (which is just a highly electrically damaged group of cells) is the almost guaranteed result of a diet of processed and electrically distorted foods. If we graphed the increase in cancer in our population and superimposed this on a graph showing the increase of manufactured, preserved, and chemically laced foods, those graphs, I suggest, would resemble each other.

We have been struggling with ever-increasing levels of degenerative diseases for the last number of years, and now with the dawn of the new millennium, we have available to us an exciting new concept to embrace. That of an electrical universe, a universe where everything is connected, and this connectivity is fundamental in supporting the life of everything else. If we use these concepts in the way we grow and prepare our food and nutritional support, I believe we can look forward to an amazingly healthy life. This fundamental concept is the change of consciousness we have all been searching for. This can and will lead us to fulfilling our desires and dreams.

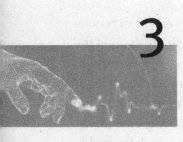

3

The Problems with Vegetarianism

One issue that arises frequently when I explain nutrition to others is that of vegetarianism, which many people today believe is a healthy approach to eating. Vegetarianism is the practice of following a meat-free diet. Veganism, a type of vegetarianism, involves the elimination of eggs, milk, cheese, or any animal products at all from the diet. There are many books, theories, and beliefs that extol the supposed benefits of vegetarianism. Many readers may find themselves surprised by electrical nutrition's take on vegetarianism.

In the already vigorous debate between vegetarians and nonvegetarians, it is obvious that the concepts of electrical nutrition discussed in earlier chapters will open up a whole new argument.

SYMPTOMS OF VEGETARIANISM

I have thousands of former vegetarians among my clients. Time and again I am amazed by the consistent pattern of malnourishment of the vegetarians I see. It is frighteningly clear to me each time an ardent vegetarian walks into my clinic. They are generally quiet-spoken, listless, and totally lacking in vitality and passion. One woman in particular comes to mind. Her complexion was incredibly pale, and she looked as if there were no meat on her bones. It was as if she were being eaten up from the inside out and all her energy was depleted by her body's attempts at survival without adequate nutritional backup. She was using up all her reserves and mining her body. She typifies the many young vegetarians who look just as unhealthy as overweight fast-food, armchair sports addicts, if not more so. Neither has a balanced understanding of nutrition.

This condition, sadly, is typical of the long-term vegetarians I have seen over the last fifteen years as part of my natural health practice. It was this startling reality that inspired me to question our entire nutritional understanding. People were coming to me at what should have been the prime of their lives—twenty to thirty years old—who had been strict vegetarians for ten or more years, and their bodies were literally falling apart.

At first, this shocked me. Then, when I questioned my vegetarian patients, I noticed a familiar pattern emerging. When they first became vegetarians, these people noticed some improvement in their health, vigor, and vitality, which made them ardent believers in vegetarianism. Then, after five years or so on a strict vegetarian diet, their vitality started to drop. After ten years on a vegetarian diet, chronic malnutrition started to manifest itself in multiple areas. Entire systems were starting to shut down.

Some of the symptoms of vegetarianism that have become very easy for me to recognize are extreme paleness, suggesting a lack of iron; lack of skin tone and deep sunken eyes, which signify major mineral deficiencies; dark areas immediately under the eyes, signifying liver and kidney stress; and, often, chronic low vitality that manifests itself as extremely low to no libido in the males and irregular or absent menstrual periods in women, coupled with severe conception difficulties.

Among the symptoms most complained of among vegetarians are digestive disorders. If a client mentions digestive problems, my immediate response now is to ask if he or she is a vegetarian. In fact, I am generally about 99-percent accurate when identifying vegetarians solely on the basis of their symptoms of malnutrition. Put plainly, I can pick 'em a mile off.

Gynecological problems are also common in vegetarians. Low protein intake contributes to inability to conceive as well as other problems. When young women come to me with reproductive system problems, usually manifested in their inability to conceive, I always tell them that they will continue to have difficulty in keeping their bodies working if they continue to follow their vegetarian diet. I could do only so much for them—I would be treating only the symptoms and not the cause. The cause could well be malnutrition with severe protein deficiency.

Protein deficiency and mineral depletion, coupled with chronic low levels of vitality, are rampant among the vegetarians of the Western Hemisphere. More than 90 percent of vegetarians who have come to me because of an inability to conceive have had their conception problems solved by reconstructing the damaged electrical circuitry of the reproductive system and by dramatically increasing their protein intake, usually in the form of red meat.

I have found in my clinic that emotional imbalances in many young girls can be dramatically reduced by taking the grain out of their diet and increasing the protein, particularly red meat. Adequate levels of protein also assist in the production of antibodies, which helps build the immune response.

Let me add that I also know vegetarians who understand the necessity of maintaining adequate levels of protein in the body and are very conscientious in making sure they take in enough protein daily. Those vegetarians who are informed and aware of their bodies' needs for adequate protein intake do not suffer from the disadvantages of a meat-free, protein-deficient diet (though they may still suffer from B-vitamin and iron deficiencies). They have generally realized early on that grain is not good for them and have eliminated it from their diet. However, there is only a handful of these healthy vegetarians.

I chuckle to myself when I recall a good friend telling me that she would not have a vegetarian lover because they do not have enough "chi" (life-force energy). "They are all poor lovers . . . weak, low-energy men" (her words, not mine). This, of course, may or may not be true; however, the story gets even funnier, because my friend is a strict vegetarian herself. In my clinical experience, it seems that the above story is an accurate depiction of many vegetarian men. Either the men themselves have visited me with health issues such as inability to maintain an erection, lack of sex drive, or prostate problems, or it has been their wives or partners who have divulged this information. It seems that sexual function is directly relative to the level of protein in one's diet.

ALIVE FOODS

There is a theory that raw vegetables are healthiest because they are still "alive." From an energy perspective, everything is alive. Everything you can see, feel, or touch transmits a frequency of energy, otherwise you would not be able to perceive it, nor would we be able to photograph it. Even when something is considered "dead" from a normally held perception, in essence it is still "alive" energetically because it is still transmitting energy. This is a difficult concept to understand, but it is the basis of modern quantum physics.

The only way anything survives on this earth is by taking the vibratory rate of another and absorbing it as part of itself. Nothing survives without this ingestion of other living things. Thus, the theory that vegetables are better for you because they are alive when you eat them and that animal flesh is not good for you because it is dead, is based on an incorrect premise. Life is not defined only by whether or not something is running around. If it were, all fruit and vegetables would be dead, which is obviously not the case. How alive something is can be measured by whether it is tied to the ground by roots or evolved enough to be running around as an animal. As discussed earlier, the aliveness of different food sources can also be indexed to the speed with which it rots/ferments (the Rock-to-Rot theory).

Vegetarians often tell me that they do not eat meat because they do not want to kill an animal, unaware that spirulina, a common vegetarian protein source, is, in essence, thousands of microscopic "critters." (Blue-green algae are sometimes referred to as "animal" because of their likeness in many respects to the creatures of the animal kingdom. Their flesh is protein, and they are definitely very much alive).

So is it okay to kill if we cannot see it? Is it okay to kill something whose death is not observable to us, but not an animal because their dying is more obvious? To me that is like a little child hiding in the corner with hands covering his eyes, thinking nobody can see him!

Aliveness can readily be quantified by a substance's vibratory rate—the frequency that is contained within its atomic structure. The vibratory rate of a substance can be determined by measuring the amount of time it takes to start decaying. As we all know, animal protein starts to decay much faster than vegetative matter. The less life force (aliveness) there is, the more slowly things decay (closer to the rock frequency). The more life force (aliveness) there is, the more quickly they decay (farther away from the rock frequency).

THE TRANSFER OF ENERGY FROM FOOD TO HUMANS

There is no living plant or animal on earth that does not obtain its nourishment from another plant or animal; so in essence there is no death—only one life form becoming another. It is essentially a process of a continuous transformation of energy. The taking of life from another is the natural process of this continuous energy (nourishment) transfer here on earth.

One of the arguments put forward by proponents of vegetarianism is that in the taking of the life of an animal for our nutrition, any negative energy resulting from the trauma or fear felt by the animal during slaughter can be transferred to us in the subsequent food. The eating of vegetables, they claim, lessens the possibility of taking on this fear energy. A good argument, until we realize that all life—plant and animal—is energy, and all energy contains a consciousness and is affected by its environment. Is it not possible, then, that the plant may also be traumatized and hold within its energy field traumatic and fearful energy resulting from being cut or pulled from its connection with the soil—its connection with what was its lifeline?

The suggestion by proponents of vegetarianism is that very few animals are slaughtered in an honorable way and these animals' flesh could contain trauma and fear frequencies in their flesh. However, the same argument can be used in the case of the modern way of harvesting fruit and vegetables. Just imagine the trauma and fear that a grain of wheat or rice must feel as it is devoured by a huge noisy machine called a combine harvester. The plant is cut off at the stem, fed into a spinning drum, and spun around at high speed, hitting metal teeth that thrash off the grain. The grain is then dragged up (by means of a large screw inside a tube) so it can crash down into a holding hopper in the bowels of the machine. Beaten and thrashed (that's what these machines used to be called—"thrashers"), the energy fields that surround and are contained in the grain are literally beaten to destruction (and we haven't even looked at the trauma and fear the grain goes through by being smashed into a million pieces in the milling and grinding process). And does fruit fare any better? Many fruit orchards are harvested with machines that grip the trees with great vice-like grippers that violently shake the tree until all the fruit is torn off the branches. Absolute terror for the fruit, I'm sure. Most modern harvesting of fruit and vegetables is carried out with similar energy-damaging and physically abusive mechanical means.

Giving Honor—a Positive Energy Transfer

Just as the slaughtering of an animal needs to be done with reverence and honor, so too we need to harvest fruits and vegetables with the same reverence and honor. Everything is a vibrating frequency of energy, everything contains a consciousness, everything is alive.

Most traditional cultures slaughtered and harvested with ceremony; in fact, the biggest and most sacred ceremonies were always associated with either a hunting expedition or harvest. In New Zealand and Australia, there are tens of thousands of sheep slaughtered in large slaughterhouses with individual ceremonial ritual and prayers of thanks for each animal, given by an attending holy person. This is carried out so that these animals can be exported to countries that require slaughtering in the presence of a holy person. The honoring and blessing of food and its source has a powerful effect on normalizing any disharmonic frequencies that maybe contained within it.

In a community in Scotland called Findhorn, members discovered that words, or even thoughts of thanks directed to a carrot, for example, before it was pulled from the ground, enabled the carrot to maintain almost the same harmonious energy it had when it was still growing. You see, it is not the taking of another life for our nourishment that is the issue, but rather the honor, or lack of honor, we give to that life.

Grasping the concept that our thoughts, words or intentions can change the subtle frequencies of energy in plant or animal tissue is a big step for many. Fortunately we have researchers such as Dr. Lee H. Lorenzen, biochemist from the United States, and Masaru Emoto, president of IHM Research Institute in Japan, who together have taken the understanding of the consciousness of life to the forefront of modern science.[1] They have shown that thoughts and spoken words around, or even a written word placed against a container of water effect measurable changes of frequency within the water. Apparently the energy contained in the writing was enough to affect the water.

The water researchers were able to show the change in frequency by photographing the water in a crystalline formation immediately before the frozen water became liquid. The photographs, taken with a magnetic resonance analyzer (MRA) equipped with a powerful microscope and camera, showed that the shape and complexities of the crystals changed radically with different thoughts and words. Feelings and words of love made complex and beautiful crystal shapes, and negative feelings or words broke up the crystal formations. Environmental pollution had similar effects on the shapes. The differing crystal shapes represented the different frequencies being picked up by the water and influencing its electrical matrix, which changed its structure and shape.

If water can be influenced by the subtle energy frequencies of thoughts and words, then surely so can plants and animals (and our food), which most of us would perceive as having a greater or higher consciousness (frequency) than water. It also should be noted that our bodies, animals, most plants, and the earth's surface all contain approximately 70 percent water—so our thoughts, feelings and words affect everything. Honor to everything, and everything with honor.

Regardless of any trauma that may or may not have been infused into the plant or animal at the time of slaughtering or harvesting, it is possible for us to bring the food into harmony by saying grace or blessing the food before eating. The water researchers mentioned above have shown that this transmission of our honoring thoughts has a very real and measurable impact. Perhaps this is all that is required to harmonize any traumatic frequencies.

WE ARE DESIGNED FOR MEAT-EATING

Another argument made in favor of vegetarianism is that the intestinal tract of humans is too long to allow animal protein to pass through in a timely manner. The theory holds that because of the length of our intestinal tract, meat becomes putrid in our bowels. The flaw here is that this argument was made in comparing the length of the human gastrointestinal tract to that of dogs.[2] Considering the many differences between dogs and humans, it is clear that this comparison is faulty.

In fact, if our digestive processes are working harmoniously, with the necessary enzymes, bacteria, and all the other parameters operating correctly, it is impossible for any food to become putrid in our bowels. Putrification is the result of improper fermentation, mostly caused by incorrect food combining. The length of the gastrointestinal tract governs how much time the body has to extract the nutrients from the food—it has nothing to do with putrification. Our intestinal tract length is perfect for the extraction of the nutrients from fast-fermenting meat and other animal protein and just long enough to handle the slower fermenting and nutrient release of some vegetation.

Grains, however, are another story. Nature made them to be largely unrottable, and their stored nutrients and life energy were never designed to be released by fermentation. Grains have to survive without decaying when buried under snow, washed away in a flood, buried in mud, and blown by the wind to land on the wet soil. Months later in the spring, when the soil temperature and sunlight hours are right, the seeds germinate and sprout into grass to feed the animals and their young. They have to be quite hardy to endure all of the assaults thrown their way.

Herbivorous animals, such as cows and sheep, have much longer digestive tracts than ours because of the extreme difficulty inherent in extracting nutrients from slowly fermenting vegetation. Cows regurgitate their food to grind it yet again (a process known as chewing their cud) in order to break open the cellulose wall of the plant cell so that fermentation can be facilitated. More than 80 percent of a cow's energy gets used up in the process of digesting the plant-based food. Only 20 percent of the energy she extracts from the food is available for production (making milk) and her life-support systems. On the other hand, a dog, which is a carnivore, has an extremely short digestive tract that is perfectly capable of digesting fast-fermenting meat and extracting its nutrients but has difficulty digesting vegetable matter properly.

A dog's input/usage ratio is far greater than that of a cow. A dog uses only 20 percent of its energy in the digestive process because flesh is so easy to ferment. (That is why farm dogs can run and run all day on a bit of raw meat and a bone to chew at night to extract the marrow from). Remember the life-force availability inherent in the Rock-to-Rot theory discussed previously.

Humans have been ingesting animal protein since day one. We evolved eating animal protein (remember the "hunter" in the hunter-gatherer), and we are still here. Fish and meat (particularly red meat) also give us more nutrients, more minerals, and more energy in exchange for less work by our digestive system than any other known food source. The most complete and readily available source of the building blocks of life and vitality are contained in flesh.

Many of the old cultures had extremely healthy and disease-free bodies despite eating large portions of animal protein, as has been made clear by the extensive studies of Dr. Weston Price, who studied the health of the Swiss, Gaelic, Eskimo, North American Indians, Polynesians, several tribes of Africa, Australian Aborigines, Torres Strait Islanders, New Zealand Maori, and Peruvian Indians.[3] Animal protein is a far more easily digested food, and its nutrient extraction is far more efficient than that of vegetation. Humans, with their medium-length intestinal tract (we are omnivores, eating a 20-percent herbivorous and 80-percent carnivorous diet), have the ability to extract all the nutrients from quick-fermenting flesh but only a small percentage of the nutrients from the slow-fermenting grains and other vegetative matter.

That humans do not have long incisor teeth like canines is often offered as evidence that we were not meant to be meat-eaters. In fact, incisor teeth are not a requirement for the chewing or digesting of flesh. Our flat, grinding teeth and sideways-flexing jaw are more than capable of easily crushing and breaking open the cellular structure of flesh, which is far easier to do than breaking open the cellular structure of vegetative matter. (Remember that the cow has to have two or three goes at grinding up vegetative matter).

The only reason canines have incisor teeth is that they have to kill with their mouths. I have yet to see a canine proficient with a bow and arrow or a gun. To pierce the thick hide and expose the jugular vein to make the kill, incisor teeth are necessary. They are not used for the actual chewing of flesh.

HUMANS HAVE BEEN MEAT-EATERS SINCE TIME IMMEMORIAL

As I said earlier, humans have always been a race of hunter-gatherers—primarily of hunters. The mainstay of the diet was always meat. The "gathered" food merely supplemented the meat. Once game started to dwindle, whole communities sometimes had to move on in search of new prey or risk perishing.

Historic records show that one of the healthiest groups of modern people, before the intrusion of Western foods, were the Inuit people of northern Canada. Their diet consisted mostly of meat and fish, generally consumed raw. This diet furnished all of the nutrients essential for health, including a good supply of B vitamins, some vitamin C, and vitamins A and D.[4] According to Vilhjalmur Stefansson, the intrusion of Western foods into Inuit society began during the nineteenth century when whalers traded their preserved foods—predominantly flour, tea, and sugar—to the Inuit in exchange for fresh meat.[5] Most of the ancient cultures ate their meat and fish raw, which contributed greatly to their well-being. The heating of foods, especially of animal protein, destroys many of the nutrients and enzymes required for proper digestion.[6] The powerful bodies of the tribes of Africa and the amazing physiques of the Pacific Island peoples (prior to the arrival of "civilization" and our unnatural foods) were all developed with a predominance of animal or fish protein in the diet.

All the earliest humans were hunters who also gathered fruit, berries, and small amounts of seeds (grain) to store for times of food shortage. They were never farmers. Farming in the modern sense started only in the 1800s when the American John Deere manufactured the first steel plow. Before that it was almost impossible to plow any great area to grow grain.

Degenerative diseases, including cancer, were largely unheard of, yet many people living at the time had a life expectancy not too different from the present. There are many records, including the Bible, that suggest that some old cultures had far greater life expectancies with their hunting and gathering than we enjoy today.

It is simply untrue to suggest that the human intestinal tract cannot safely digest animal protein. We evolved to the top of the food chain by eating animal protein. We became the most evolved by eating food with the the highest vibratory rate. To clearly see the importance of animals as food we only have to look back less than 200 years to a time when poaching (hunting or stealing an animal from somebody else's land) carried a penalty more severe than murder. Even in biblical times, wealth was measured by the number of goats or sheep one owned. They supplied the fiber for clothing and the protein for nourishment, two very valuable commodities.

THE HUMAN BODY NEEDS PROTEIN

The human body can extract its life force, its vitality, only from its nutritional intake. Children, as well as menstruating and breastfeeding women, require high levels of protein to maintain their full vigor.

Protein is the main tissue builder of the body and is the basic substance of every cell, including muscles, bone, blood, skin, nails, hair, and internal organs, hence the necessity for maintaining adequate levels of protein in our diet. Protein is essential for enzyme production, which enables the electrical processes to take place. It is also important for the production of hormones that regulate and control bodily functions, including emotional stability.

We all have to make choices of which food offers us the most life-giving nutrition. Our bodies can draw energy only from the food that evolved with us in nature. It must contain nature's electrical matrix to be available to us. Our bodies can only recognize food as food if it can electrically connect with it using the processes that have been laid down by nature over billions of years. To think we can change food by processing and preserving it and still have it be electrically available to us is to have eyes that will not see. Likewise, to hold that vegetative matter is a better choice to give our bodies the best chance of a disease-free and vibrant life is to ignore the very basic facts of who we are, where we come from, how nature works, and what our place in it is. Belief structures are very hard to change, and we often base our identity on what we believe. To change our beliefs can often leave us without an identity, which can be very scary for most of us; however, when presented with a logic that is so clear that you cannot deny its truth, you may slowly be able to mold your beliefs to see a different truth.

We are not aliens from another place. Our bodies evolved here on earth, and to have healthy bodies, we need to feed them electrically recognizable food—food the way nature made it. Healthy bodies also require food that is the highest on the evolutionary ladder and that contains the highest vibratory rate. Animal protein has the highest vibratory rate and contains the greatest amount of life force—life force that becomes us when eaten. Animal and fish protein gives us the highest return in energy availability, followed closely by raw fresh fruit and berries. Then come green leafy vegetables, followed by the root crops and other more solid vegetables. Grains are the lowest. To advocate a predominantly vegetarian diet could unwittingly deprive people of the best-quality, highest-vibratory-rate foods. Even the Dalai Lama, who is considered to be one of the most spiritual people on earth, understands his body's requirements for meat and eats it regularly ever since falling ill with hepatitis in 1967.[7] His doctors felt that the lack of meat in his diet was a cause of his ailing health. After two years of vegetarianism, the Dalai Lama returned to his prior eating habits, and his health improved.

A Note on Juicing

Juicing of fruits and vegetables is very popular among vegetarians, and the natural-foods set; however, this practice dramatically alters the electrical matrix and results in food that is no longer in the form nature intended. I have personally seen the development of toxic effects from an overdose of juiced vegetables taken in by people who believed they were living very healthily. Your digestive tract was never intended to absorb excessive amounts of twentieth-century juicing technology. Sometimes too much juicing results in diarrhea, which is a symptom of an extremely stressed and agitated digestive tract—not a desirable state to be in.

It should also be noted that juicing and putting the fruits and vegetables through the blender is a homogenization process, and we are all aware of the arguments surrounding homogenized milk and how bad that is. Homogenization, in essence, is the breaking apart of the molecular structure, and your high-speed blender has a cutter that ro-

tates at approximately 30,000 revolutions per minute. The perfect ho-
mogenizer—total destruction to the molecular structure and the energy fields surrounding it.

However, in severe life-threatening disease states, such as cancer
and liver failure, juicing is advantageous because it fractures the cellulose of the cell walls of the food, making the food molecules more easily accessible to the body. This lowers the amount of energy required
for digestion, freeing energy to be used to assist the body in its recovery
process.

SUMMARY

Vegetarianism may not be as healthy as was once thought, especially
when we understand the electrical process of digestion, as outlined in
Chapter 2. The body needs available sources of protein in order to
function at the highest vibratory rate possible. Protein is required to
maintain our health and well-being—without it we may suffer many
serious electrical malfunctions. Symptoms of vegetarianism are outlined, and in the next chapter we detail the various types of protein and
their electrical availability so that you can make informed choices, with
the understanding that those choices affect your energy levels and overall health. The choice is ultimately yours, and we provide this information so that you can make an educated choice.

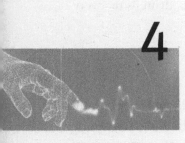

4

The Electrical Availability of Foods

Understanding and accepting the need for protein leads us to ask more questions regarding the quality and source of our protein and to question whether all protein is of the same electrical value. For instance, consumers often automatically purchase chicken in the belief that they are getting a healthier product than they would if they bought red meat. This is not always the case. To help you understand why this is not the case and to answer other questions about the electrical value of proteins, we need to explore in some depth farming and production methods so that you can be better informed regarding dietary issues. We will also discuss problems that arise in connection with our consumption of vegetables, fruits, and grains.

To make educated choices regarding which protein foods to eat, it is important to realize that the way animals are raised has a direct impact on the electrical quality of the food derived from them (also pertinent to vegetable growing). For the highest electrical, and therefore nutritional, value, the goal is to choose food from animals that were both raised and slaughtered in the most honorable and humane way, as is the case with organic farming methods and other production systems that I will explain as we move through this chapter.

BEEF

Many people believe that red meat, particularly beef, is a less healthy meat option because it contains high levels of antibiotics and hormones. Let us look at the normal meat-raising process. A calf starts off its life freely foraging on the range country or confined in outside feedlots. It stays with its mother for approximately six to nine months and then is weaned onto grass if it is raised on the range or onto alfalfa hay and corn silage if it is a feedlot-reared calf. The range cattle at approximately ten months of age are brought into the feedlot and then fed the same diet as the feedlot-reared stock for another three months or so.

At approximately thirteen months of age, the cow or steer is considered to be prime. It is then slaughtered, and its meat is used for prime cuts and steaks. This meat is practically hormone free, antibiotic free, and unaltered in any way. This is even more so in New Zealand and Australia, as all the cattle are raised outside with little other factors than green grass and sunshine.

Young cattle are incredibly hardy animals and, unlike commercially produced chickens, cattle in North America are raised predominantly outside. Cattle feed consists of either range grass or, in the case of the feedlots, top-quality alfalfa hay and corn silage, both of which require far fewer chemicals in their production than do wheat or barley (the normal feed stock for chickens).

The beef cattle finishing industry, which produces our prime beef, is at the top end of the food production squeaky-clean scale. This is particularly true for meat with the "Certified Angus" mark. However, the lower-grade beef that is made into ground beef, hamburger, sausages, and beef products other than prime cuts comes predominantly from old dairy cows that have come to the end of their milk-producing years and bulls (older male cattle).

Dairy cows, which are housed lactating animals, are machine-milked twice a day. This can make them very susceptible to udder infections, which may require antibiotic treatment. However, milk from an antibiotic-treated cow is never intentionally supplied to milk-processing factories because this is illegal. Milk supplied to processing plants is tested daily, and penalties for supplying antibiotic-contaminated milk are extremely severe.

At times in the past, dairy cows were fed with a natural hormone to increase their milk production. This increases milk levels only fractionally because of the physical constraints of the cows' udder capacity. Farmers are not stupid—to overstimulate a cow's milk production is detrimental to the cow's health and thereby to the farmer's profitability. However, a European ban on beef and dairy products containing any traces of the recombinant bovine growth hormone has brought to the American agricultural industry's attention the worldwide concern about foods containing non-naturally occurring hormones. New Zealand and Australia, like Europe, have always had hormone-free dairy industries.

Since antibiotics and hormones can stay in all flesh for quite some time, there have always been very strict holding periods between antibiotic or hormone use and slaughter in the beef and dairy industries. There are very strict controls and testing for antibiotic residues in the dairy and beef industries, so despite some bad press to the contrary, the hormone and antibiotic levels that prevail in the dairy and beef industry are much lower than most people think. The meat to avoid if you are concerned about antibiotics and hormones would be ground beef, as that is where the meat from old dairy cows and bulls that were given female hormones to calm them down is used. Purchasing the more expensive cuts of meat ensures that you are getting a clean, top-quality product. Farming is all about having healthy animals. There is no profitability in having sick cows that need medication.

Many people are often under the misconception that low-fat cuts of meats are preferable for a healthy diet. However, when we look at the science of nutrition, despite a multitude of publications to the contrary, it becomes abundantly clear that fat does not make you fat. In essence, enzymatic and liver activity converts all food in the body into the essential fatty acids needed to fire the electrical spark mentioned earlier. Animal fats require very little processing in order to be converted into essential fatty acids. I once again refer to the healthy Inuit people and their natural diet of seal blubber, which, in essence, is straight fat. In their natural habitat, this fat was eaten raw (just the way nature made it). Nature does not produce any animal protein without fat in it. Whether you look at milk (including mother's milk), eggs, or meat (from all animals), they all contain fat. Modern nutritionists who advocate a fat-reduced or fat-free diet are suggesting that nature, in her billion of years of evolution and wisdom, got it wrong.

Another reason for eating red meat is that it supplies more amino acids, more iron, more B vitamins, and more zinc and other minerals in the perfect ratio for uptake by our bodies than any other known food. In fact, red meat has been consumed by the human race since we evolved on this earth. It has always been the most revered and honored food source.

LAMB

Correctly graded lamb from New Zealand or Australia would be even better than some prime beef, as these animals never see anything except their mothers' milk, natural green grass, and the joy of life. Sadly, it is difficult to purchase genuine lamb (a young sheep less than nine months of age) in the continental United States. The grading system (or lack thereof) for sheep meat in the United States often does not distinguish between young and old sheep. When you purchase American "lamb," it could be meat from an old ewe (old female sheep with meat as tough as old boots and a smell to match). Everywhere else in the world, such meat would be graded as mutton. Real "lamb" is a specifically defined age and weight specification that can be relied on if the meat comes from New Zealand or Australia. It is arguably the purest and environmentally cleanest meat source produced anywhere in the world.

CHICKEN

Chicken is not necessarily a healthier option than red meat. Most chicken available in supermarkets is a product of commercial chicken farming, usually a highly sophisticated, extremely regimented battery-farming operation—the birds are caged and fed an artificially formulated diet that sometimes contains antibiotics as standard ingredients. The antibiotics are often considered necessary because of the chronic disease potential created by the crammed cages the chickens live in.

Modern hens have been bred to have an astonishingly fast growth rate for a few weeks, often achieved with the assistance of growth hormones that are added to their feed ration. They are slaughtered at a very young age (approximately sixteen to eighteen weeks) before chronic disease has time to manifest. If they are left to grow to the desired weight without growth hormone, the death rate due to disease increases dramatically. In fact, part of the reason the chickens have to be forced to reach a desired weight sooner is that so many chickens would die if left to live a normal life span that the farmer would wind up losing tons of money. This death rate is brought on by the extremely crowded conditions the chickens are forced to live in.

The hens never see sunlight, and because of forced growth they are extremely anemic. In no way does their flesh carry within it the correct electrical matrix to give us the nutrition we expect. This is a very different animal from the one Grandma served for Sunday dinner when we were kids. The packaged chicken from the supermarket may be an electrically distorted, genetically altered, hormonally treated, force-fed, antibiotic-laced, deficient form of protein. But it looks nice. The same applies to much of the commercially raised turkey and other fowl.

However, free-range or organically produced chickens are a wonderful protein source. Be aware of advertisements claiming that the chickens are fed a vegetarian diet. Chickens are carnivorous (in their natural habitat, they eat bugs, slugs, worms, and anything else that moves that they can catch) and to feed them an artificial vegetarian diet is definitely not the way nature intended.

Free-range organic fertilized eggs are also a wonderful source of protein. Eggs that come from hens that are free to run around outside and that have been allowed to be fertilized by the male are a very powerful source of protein. It should be noted here that hens are not vegetarians, so be wary of egg sources that state the hens have been fed a vegetarian diet or a diet high in soy.

DAIRY PRODUCTS

Milk, cheese, yogurt, and butter are wonderful sources of protein. However, the fermentation of dairy products in our digestive tract is severely compromised with pasteurization. Raw (nonheated) dairy products are far superior to high-temperature-pasteurized processed dairy foods. If you can obtain raw (unheated) milk, raw butter, and no-added-sugar whole-milk yogurt, your stomach will stand a much better chance of extracting nature's gifts.

Many times in my clinic, I have been asked questions about lactose intolerance (difficulty digesting dairy products). I answer these questions by saying that technically there is no such thing as dairy intolerance. Lactose intolerance simply means the body is low on the important lactase digestive enzyme. With adequate supplementation of digestive enzymes that include lactase, dairy intolerance can be alleviated.

The fats in milk, butter, and cream are among the most beneficial protein sources available to the human body not only supplying important protein but also assisting to clean and heal the digestive tract. As it is "protein the way nature made it," dairy fat does not make you fat—it is pure life-giving energy.

Three billion years of evolution put fat in all milk (including breast milk); those who choose low-fat or nonfat milk and dairy products must be suggesting that nature got it wrong. I suggest that the logic in making this choice is the error. Nature never got it wrong; the fat molecule in dairy products is one of the most pure, essential forms of protein available to the human body. The value of dairy products is the reason why the humble cow is the oldest-known domesticated animal on earth. She gave us the calf and she milks for ten months of the year. Whole-milk yogurt and cheese (particularly European-style cheeses that contain no food colorings or chemical additives) have already gone through part of the fermentation process because of the bacterial and enzymatic action that converted them into yogurt and cheese; these are very available sources of protein for the body. Once again, keep it whole (with the fat in), and if possible, choose organically produced raw dairy products.

BEANS AND NUTS

Yes, there are sources of protein other than animal products. Beans and nuts are two common such sources.

Beans are relatively hard to digest and tend to cause gas; however, they are good sources of protein when prepared correctly. In some older cultures, beans were fermented in goat, sheep, or breast milk for a few days so the natural enzymes in the milk could break down the protein in the beans to make them more easily assimilable when eaten. This was also the case with many varieties of nuts.

I will never forget the time when my children were young and I had the opportunity to look after them for a weekend. My wife at the time had prepared a large pot of bean salad so that the "kids wouldn't starve when she was away," insinuating (rightly so!) that I, not being "the man about the house," would probably let the kids starve or just raid the freezer for all the ice cream. However, her act of concern fell rather flat (no pun intended) when all of us nearly died from toxic food poisoning—true story! Nobody had told my dear wife that you had to soak and drain kidney beans repeatedly to get all the toxins out of them. The incredible-tasting bean salad was 70-percent raw, unsoaked kidney beans, and by early Sunday morning, the three kids and I were in no condition to fend for ourselves, let alone each other. My wife had arranged to have a neighbor check on us, and on Sunday morning she found three very sick kids and one very blurry-eyed "not-a-man-about-the-house" struggling to clean up the results of three kids not having the strength to make it to the bathroom in time. This is still a family joke when the kids (now all grown up and healthy) come together for family gatherings. It is known as "the day Mom tried to kill us." I didn't go near kidney beans for years after that little intestinal tract clean-out.

Though nuts are good sources of protein, they do not ferment at all well. In fact, nature made nuts, which are the seedpods of trees, to be largely unfermentable, not unlike the seeds of the grasses like wheat and barley. This is why squirrels and the like can store nuts to be used as winter rations. Dried nuts like those we get from our supermarket were never eaten in times of old without being prefermented in milk or water. To ingest dried nuts is to largely waste a very good protein source. They do not give up their electrical energy in the short time our digestive system has to process food.

In parts of southern Europe, nut protein is eaten in higher quantities than meat. In Turkey, for instance, there are many hundreds of dishes based on chestnuts, a common protein eaten in that part of the world. However, the nuts are very seldom eaten dry but are prefermented—sometimes for days before being cooked—and then eaten. On the rock-to-rot scale, nuts do not fare too well, and vegetarians who rely on dried nuts for their protein can develop nutritional deficiencies.

Spirulina

Another popular protein source is spirulina (blue-green algae). It is easily digested and quickly assimilated and is an excellent source of vitamins, amino acids, and absorbable iron. It is especially good for menstruating women and breastfeeding mothers. If you choose to use spirulina as a protein source, search for an organically produced product, as this will be more electrically available to your body.

Spirulina could be considered a better protein source than beans or nuts as it is more easily fermented; however, to obtain adequate levels of protein from spirulina, the required intake would be prohibitively expensive compared to red meat.

Phytonutrients

A completely vegetarian, electrically available source of amino acids and B group vitamins can be found in a plant-based source of nutrition (sometimes referred to as phytonutrients). This is basically the energy component of the plant that the body would normally extract through digestion. When taken in large doses, these nutrients can feed and nourish the body to some extent and can be used by vegetarians to alleviate some of the chronic protein and other deficiencies that many have. So, *yes* there may be help for ardent vegetarians who want to integrate electrical nutrition into their way of life.

Tocotrienols, in essence the molecule that vitamin E is extracted from, are the components of plant cells that the body converts into available protein and then to essential fatty acids. Modern nutritional science extracts these components from plant sources amd combines them with digestive enzymes so the body has access to the naturally occurring B vitamins and amino acids. There are some extraordinarily good electrically formulated tocotrienol-based supplements on the market today. This is very high-tech and relatively new supplement formulation technology and should not be overlooked by anyone seeking a very powerful nutritional supplement. Some of the better formulations, from an electrical point of view, are those from Avena Originals and the Electrical Nutrition Professional Company. These high-tech electrically formulated products are not available through normal retail avenues. They are sold exclusively to health professionals and some member-only network marketing companies. See Appendix A for information on how your health-care practitioner can obtain these products.

POOR PROTEIN CHOICES

Just because you are eating protein-rich foods does not necessarily mean those foods are good for you. Some protein sources simply are not electrically available to the body. Read on to learn about sources of protein that you should be wary of.

Pork

It appears that pork has a relatively low electrical interface with our bodies. Hunted wild hogs seem to contain an electrical matrix that is more compatible with the human body. The raising techniques of farm-raised hogs, which include a high-grain diet (not their natural diet), seems to have a detrimental effect on the electrical availability of their meat. It could also be said that hogs are highly intelligent and emotionally sensitive, and their confinement in modern farming environments can have a huge impact that reflects on the frequency contained in their flesh. In comparison, cattle are incredibly docile animals, and their life-force energies do not seem to be affected by their raising environments to the same level as hogs'.

In addition, a large proportion of what Americans see in their supermarkets as pork or bacon would be condemned to the blood-and-bone fertilizer plants in most other Western countries. Most Americans do not know what quality bacon looks like.

Hog farmers in the United States get paid per pound of live weight. By comparison, in Canada, New Zealand, Australia, and England, farmers are financially *penalized* if their hogs weigh more than a certain figure. Farmers are also penalized if the hogs' percentage of fat is over the allowable limit. Quality gets rewarded and quantity gets penalized. In the United States, the opposite seems to be the case. In addition, most commercially produced ham and bacon contain high levels of preservatives such as nitrates, which inhibit the digestive process.

If you do choose pork as a protein source, look for organically raised pork.

Soy Products

Tofu and soymilk are products made from soybeans, and many people believe them to be excellent sources of protein and other nutrients. Soy is especially popular among vegetarians. Unfortunately, once again, we find that conventional wisdom may well be somewhat in error. In fact, tofu and soymilk are among the most highly processed, electrically damaged forms of protein we could possibly eat. Their manufacturing requires the stripping and recombining of the molecular structure of the soybean.

The electrical matrix of commercial soy products is completely foreign to our bodies. Nature does not produce tofu or soymilk; therefore, they do not contain nature's electrical matrix. Home-prepared naturally fermented soy may be more electrically available. In my opinion, tofu and soy products are extremely suspect as healthy protein sources when looked at from an electrical nutrition perspective. There are a number of published papers on studies that support this. (See the soy report in Appendix C.) As far as agriculture is concerned, soy has long been known to be toxic to animals and up until recent decades was never used as a food. It was plowed into the soil as a ground conditioner, as it fixes nitrogen into the soil.

What was listed as a minor industrial crop in the 1913 Department of Agriculture handbook now covers 72 million acres of American farmland. Modern technology has enabled what was once considered a waste product to be transformed into something that upscale consumers search out. Approximately $80 million is now spent annually on what was previously sold as an extender and meat substitute to promote it as a health product that will assist in preventing heart disease, cancer, and hot flashes.

Even in Asia, soybeans were eaten only after fermentation techniques that led to the creation of tofu were discovered. However, the Chinese and Japanese never ate large quantities of tofu, as they were aware that it contained enzyme inhibitors, which block protein digestion.

A report written by Sally Fallon and Mary Enig, Ph.D., after the Third International Soy Symposium, held in Washington D.C., in November 1999 (see Appendix C), highlights the health dangers of modern soy products. It seems that modern soy products contain "anti-nutrients" and toxins that interfere with the absorption of vitamins and minerals. The authors say that enzyme inhibitors in tofu can produce serious gastric distress, as well as reduced protein digestion, and can lead to chronic deficiencies. In test animals, these inhibitors caused enlargement of the pancreas and cancer. Soybeans contain a clot-promoting substance that causes red blood cells to clump together, which can lead to strokes and other blood-clotting and artery congestive problems.

Soy also contains growth inhibitors and substances that depress thyroid function and inhibit the uptake of essential minerals such as calcium, magnesium, copper, iron, and zinc. That is why vegetarians who consume tofu run the risk of developing severe mineral deficiencies. "Zinc is called the intelligence mineral because it is needed for optimal development and functioning of the brain and nervous system," Fallon and Enig's report says. "It plays a role in protein synthesis and collagen formation; it is involved in the blood-sugar control mechanism and thus protects against diabetes; it is needed for a healthy reproductive system. Zinc is a key component in numerous vital enzymes and plays a role in the immune system. Phytates found in soy products interfere with zinc absorption more completely than with other minerals. Zinc deficiency can cause a 'spacey' feeling that some vegetarians may mistake for the high of spiritual enlightenment."

To reduce the negative effects of soy, massive processing is required. This includes mixing the soybeans with an alkaline solution and separating fibers with an acid wash—often in an aluminum tank (which leaches high levels of aluminum into the final product). The high temperatures and high pressure of the extraction processes render soy largely ineffective as a protein source. In essence, the electrical energy that was in the bean is destroyed, so processed soy products are electrically dead. Numerous flavorings, including MSG, are then added to make the processed soy edible.

Fallon and Enig's report also states that "except in times of famine, Asians consume soy products only in small amounts, as condiments, and not as a replacement for animal foods —with one exception. Celibate monks living in monasteries and leading a vegetarian lifestyle find soy foods quite helpful because they dampen libido." In women, soy intake can shut down the reproductive system and disrupt hormonal balance, which can lead to serious emotional problems, particularly among girls and menstruating women. The hot flashes that some women experience during menopause are said to be lessened by eating soy products. As soy has the effect of shutting down the reproductive system, symptoms associated with the changes that may be taking place may very well go away. The question is: Has soy fixed the perceived problem or just shut the body down somewhat? Suppressing a problem is not solving it, and suppression usually leads to further problems later.

Another startling fact presented in the report is that soy protein has received approval only as a binder in cardboard boxes. It has never achieved GRAS (generally recognized as safe) status.

As you can see, soy is clearly not a healthy alternative. I have always said that soy is an electrical time bomb, and now there is a whole host of scientific research to back this up. Just ask yourself one question when making food choices: Did nature make this food the way I am about to eat it, or has it been so highly processed and changed that my body will not be able to recognize its electrical matrix? Modern soy products are not food; they are, in essence, the protein-based glue that makes cardboard for boxes.

NUTRIENT-DEFICIENT SOILS PRODUCE NUTRIENT-DEFICIENT FOODS

Everything above the ground is a reflection of what is going on below the ground—an old farm saying that is as true today as it was a thousand years ago. All topsoil evolved from rock by way of the decay of plant material and the work of bacteria, which made available the micronutrients to the animals. As a large part of our food stems from the soil, it must then reflect its quality. If our soil is low in quality, then our food will be low in energy. In our great-grandmothers' day, every time we ate some fruit, some vegetables, or some animal protein, we got nature's bountiful basket that not only contained the evolved minerals, but also enzymes and bacteria that were living in the soil and food.

As a result of ingesting all of these components, the stomach got populated with natural bacteria and flora with every mouthful, which kept the digestion system working perfectly. The alive, healthy soil was transferred to us in most of the food we ate. Today, a large proportion of the minerals, microbacteria, and enzymes that populated the soil and food two hundred years ago do not now exist because of modern chemical farming practices, particularly in the vegetable- and fruit-growing arenas. From an electrical nutrition understanding, this is a disaster.

Back in 1936 the United States government was informed of soil nutrient problems:

The alarming fact is that foods [fruits, vegetables and grains] now being raised on millions of acres of land that no longer contains enough of certain minerals, are starving us—no matter how much we eat. No man of today can eat enough fruits and vegetables to supply his system with the minerals he requires for perfect health because his stomach isn't big enough to hold them.

The truth is that our foods vary enormously in value, and some of them aren't worth eating as food. . . . Our physical well-being is more directly dependent upon the minerals we take into our system than upon calories or vitamins or upon the precise proportions of starch, protein or carbohydrates we consume.[1]

And that was back in 1936.

Our bodies have evolved over millions of years on earth, so adaptation is an extremely slow process. Rapid change in the electrical matrix of the soil and food (as in the last hundred years or so) because of chemicals, preservatives, processing, and artificial fertilizers means that our bodies are virtually incapable of being in electrical harmony with the food we eat.

What we perceive to be nutritious is, in fact, an illusion. Wonderful-looking fruits and vegetables are not what they seem. The compatibility between the electrical matrix of the food and the electrical matrix of our bodies is out of harmony. The electrical synergy between our food and our bodies has to be correct, otherwise, food becomes a poison. This is basic electrical science. The long-term effects of ingestion of low-level poisons leads to electrical disharmony, or "disease."

In an attempt to remain economically viable and to keep the soil productive, the modern farmer often has little option other than to use chemical compounds and fertilizers. The more enlightened farmers test their soil for mineral balance and replace the necessary minerals if deficiencies occur.

One of the big distinctions between raising crops and animals is that it is very easy to have exceedingly good-looking and high-yielding crops using artificial fertilizers containing NPK (nitrogen, phosphate, and potassium) formula. Various ratios of nitrogen, phosphate, and potassium are normal fertilizer additives in modern agriculture. With this formula, the resulting crops may well have chronic mineral deficiencies, but without complex analysis, this is not apparent.

When I was in school, we germinated and grew some wheat plants in the laboratory in a container of water. Each week, we added a solution of nitrogen and, when required, phosphate and potassium. The wheat plants grew extremely well. The resulting crop, if it had been on a farmer's field, would have yielded a very high tonnage per acre. But as our agriculture science teacher informed us at the time, the mice we kept in the laboratory would have died of malnourishment if we had fed them this lovely-looking wheat because it was deficient in micronutrients and minerals. The laboratory wheat received only NPK, as do most commercially farmed crops, which does not create the full electrical matrix. In an attempt to compensate for this known deficiency in commercially produced crops, most flour is fortified with artificial nutrients, such as vitamin D. This is a far cry from anything that represents a plant grown the way nature intended. Very rarely does any cereal manufacturer, baker, or food manufacturer pay the farmer based on the mineral or micronutrient content of the crop. Normally, the farmer gets paid by the ton and can survive economically only by producing tonnage. The NPK model will produce lots of tonnage.

Farmers who raise animals have to be much more aware of micronutrient and other nutritional requirements because animals fed deficient food will very quickly show symptoms of it. Mineral and vitamin supplementation has been part of the animal-raising scene for many years. In fact, there is not a cattle farmer out there who does not know the importance of balanced nutrition. Micronutrients are top-dressed onto the land or added to the feed mix to keep the animals and soil healthy. If a farmer has a few thousand head of cattle on the ranch or in the feedlot, and the food they are given has a vitamin or mineral deficiency in it, the farmer, very quickly, will be facing a multimillion dollar catastrophe in the form of very sick and dying animals. So, even for economic reasons only, the animal production system is healthier and more balanced.

If the need for mineral supplementation has been understood in animal production for many years, why has our health system denied, and in fact, actively campaigned against the fortification of our diet in the form of mineral, herbal, and vitamin supplementation? It has often intrigued me that a can of a popular brand of cat food contains forty-two vitamin and mineral additives that are said to be essential for the healthy life of our feline friend. Yet two aisles away in the same supermarket, the jars of baby food contain only eight of the same nutritional supplements. The contents of both containers came from the same agricultural base, the same nutrient-deficient soil. Why is it that veterinary science, which was responsible for formulating the cat food, saw the importance of the micronutrient additives, while nutritionists, including doctors, do not see the same importance for our children?

Agricultural science is motivated to prevent the manifestation of disease in farm animals by its economic survival. On the other hand, the economic survival of the human medical system depends on illness (there would be little need for doctors and drugs if there was no illness). Face it, if all human diseases stopped tomorrow, there would be one tremendous hiccup in the world's financial system. If the same amount of disease that exists in humans was allowed to manifest in the farming scene, the effects on our food supply would result in mass starvation. The two health-care systems operate from opposite ends of the spectrum.

Understanding our food production system, the depletion of our soils, the mineral deficiencies in grain and vegetable production, the lack of adequate good animal protein in our diet, and our obsession with grain/sugar-based products such as bread, muffins, bagels, doughnuts, pasta, cereals, and soda, it is easy to see the reason for our rampant chronic disease. It is impossible for our bodies to function electrically in perfect harmony with the low-energy food that is our modern diet.

GRAIN—AN ELECTRICAL DRAIN

For a number of years now, the big food fad in North America has been a high-carbohydrate, grain-based diet. Many vegetarians eat a high-grain diet. While many may think they are eating healthily by following such a diet, nothing could be further from the truth. In fact, by following such a diet, they are setting themselves up for serious degenerative disorders such as chronic obesity, adult-onset diabetes, and joint degeneration, as well as emotional imbalances, reproductive system problems, and recurring yeast infections—to name just a few. (See Chapter 7 for more on this.)

When we look at modern farming practices, including the use of chemical fertilizers, artificial breeding, the manipulation of cultivars, and the use of nutrient-deficient soil, we realize that we must be producing wheat and other grains that have very little relationship to plants of even twenty years ago. Of all the crops grown, wheat is one of the most chemically sprayed and altered crops there is.

The lowering of our grain quality is largely unknown by the general populace. Due to the poor quality of our grains, the electrical matrix is far different from what it once was. Modern grains are more responsible for the accumulation of cellulite (fat) than any other food. The cellulite then holds toxins from other chemical-laced foods and in fact becomes the body's very convenient toxic waste dump.

When flour is mixed with water, it makes glue (when we were kids we made the most awesome brown-paper kites that we glued together with flour-and-water glue). Flour and sugar will clog up and destroy the human body quicker than any other food combination, including the meat-and-potato scenario.

It is frightening that a large percentage of young people in North America are fed such a diet. Their daily intake normally consists of pop, doughnuts, muffins, burgers, noodles, pasta, hot-dog buns, and various other grain- and sugar-based foods. This is the perfect recipe for obesity, endocrine system malfunction, and emotional instability, and often leads to reproductive system problems in young women—with painful and difficult periods as one of the first symptoms. Skin eruptions, acne, chronic irritability, concentration deficits, and general learning difficulties are all early manifestations of serious grain and sugar toxicity.

In our older population, obesity, lethargy, libido problems, conception problems, menopausal difficulties later in life, prostate symptoms in men, and of course the big one, joint degeneration and arthritis, are all long-term symptoms of grain toxicity and excess sugar.

Grains Do Not Rot

Looking at wheat, rye, oats, millet, and other grains from an electrical nutrition perspective, their ability to nourish the human body is relatively low, due to their low vibratory rate. If you threw some wheat (and other grain) out on the ground and waited for it to decompose, you would be waiting a long time. Yes, this process is sped up in our gastrointestinal tracts, but even then, that grain is hardly broken down before it gets eliminated. If you ingest wheat or other grains in an unground form as in whole-grain breads, rolled oats, muesli, and the like, the grain will pass through your intestinal tract largely unfermented, undigested, and completely intact.

Birds often eat whole grain (seeds) and perhaps get some nourishment from it. However, more often than not, the bird passes the undigested grain wrapped in its own fertilizer bundle. The seed is now able to germinate and grow into a new plant. This is the role of seeds in nature. It is one way nature spreads its bounty far and wide. Hens also eat grains (though in their natural habitat, they eat very little grain—their predominant food is bugs, worms, and so on—all protein. They are not vegetarians), but then again, hens carry with them their own grinding device, called a crop. Within that crop are stones, bits of glass, broken crockery if it is available, and any other very hard matter that the hen can find. She regurgitates the whole grain into this crop and grinds it. A hen can eat almost anything and digest it; in fact, the hen's digestive process is far more efficient than ours. But even with that efficiency, the hen still has to grind that grain to oblivion.

The old cultures, in times of famine, learned to grind and ferment their grains before ingesting them. It was a desperate attempt to gain some nourishment from them. Though the health-conscious may think they are making a healthful choice by eating whole grains, other than the fiber they provide to make large bowel movements, whole grains are largely useless to us nutritionally. Fiber acts like steel wool to clean our gastrointestinal tract. If we eat electrically, our "pipes" will not be clogged up, so we will no longer need the whole grains to clean us out.

Nature spent billions of years designing grain so that it gives its life force to nurture new life through the process of germination, not fermentation. In her wisdom, nature wrapped up the seed-head (grain) in a fibrous tissue and designed it to be largely unrottable. This allowed the seed the time to find just the right environment and then germinate. A seed-head can get blown away in the wind, be washed away in the flood, sit under six feet of snow, and be eaten by a bird, and still it does not rot. When germination takes place, the resulting sprout is then a complex protein, or the "flesh" of the plant. This "flesh" is now able to be fermented in an animal's digestive tract and used for growth, milk production, and vitality. This is why grazing animals have their young in the spring. There is an abundance of growing grass (protein) to supply the energy and nutritional requirements of feeding their young. In the spring there is not a seed-head to be seen in the fields; it is all green grass. There is not one grazing animal that lives on grain (seeds). The plants produced the seeds only in the fall, at the end of the growing season, when the demand for food by the animals was low. The plant can now go into its reproductive phase and drop its seed to germinate in the following spring to once again meet the demand for food by the animals.

Our digestive tract, like that of the grazing animals, is almost completely unable to ferment a seed-head (grain), whether it is whole or ground up as in flour. Nature designed the seed-head to store its life-giving energy, and when we try to eat grain, the innate frequency of the seed-head can only go into storage—in other words, lay down cellulite. The 5,000-year-old iceman found in the Otztaler Alps on the Austrian/ Italian border still had remnants of wheat in his intestinal lining. Even after 5,000 years it still had not rotted![2] That is why in agriculture to fatten up the hog or cattle, we feed them grain. Likewise, if you want to fatten up, eat grains. Grain is the hardest food to ferment and takes the most energy to digest, and we get little or nothing from it except large thighs, butts, and bellies. Remember the old farm saying: grain for gain, protein for production. From an electrical nutrition perspective, modern grains could well be considered toxic.

SUMMARY

As you can see, different food sources have different levels of electrical availability. At the top of the list would be the prime cuts of beef, New Zealand or Australian lamb, most fish, and dairy products. Organically produced sources are by far the best. Factors that compromise the body's electrical system will be outlined in the following chapters but even simply increasing your intake of electrically available protein and avoiding grains will dramatically increase your energy levels, libido, and overall well-being. Give it a go and see for yourself.

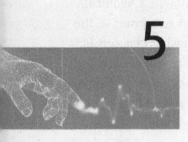

5

Assaults on the Body's
Electrical System

It could be argued that one of the most important electrical systems in the body is the immune system. If the immune system becomes compromised, then all of our bodily functions become compromised. The immune system's job is to protect the body from illness, thereby allowing the rest of the body to function properly.

Anything that compromises the body's immune system can be considered an electrical body bomb. These can include the effects of improper fermentation, doctor-prescribed medications, immunizations, recreational drugs, chemotherapy, disharmonious electromagnetic frequencies such as microwaves, aspartame (an ingredient found in most diet foods), and, believe it or not, our classic birthing model.

The immune system is electrically connected to the endocrine system. The endocrine system is a series of manufacturing plants that produce chemicals and hormones and thus set up the electrical interface for many of the body's primary functions. As the endocrine system starts to overload due to the effects of incorrect digestion and the preservatives and other additives in our food, it produces the wrong hormone at the wrong time, in the wrong amount, for the wrong reason. The resulting imbalance then affects the electrical firing of the brain cells, often inducing mood swings, anxiety, depression, chronic fatigue, PMS, and other emotional disorders. Every free radical (harmful waste product of cellular function), every piece of improperly digested food, every toxic chemical we ingest puts stress on the electrical systems of the body and produces a toxic loading on the cells.

In order to create electrical harmony, the body will look for ways to clean out the toxic buildup. It will attempt to create an environment that induces a population explosion of certain microorganisms, resulting in what we call "a cold." Getting cold at night can be a trigger for "catching a cold." Colds, however, are not actually "caught"; they are a natural correcting function arising from an imbalance within the body. This imbalance is sometimes caused by the body's drop in temperature and the resulting pH change, but more often it is caused by the body's need to lower its general toxicity—to flush the poisons out. The subsequent increase in temperature and mucus production is the body's natural way of dealing with the toxic loading. This is an electrical nutrition concept; however, there are a few scientific references that point to the importance of maintaining the correct pH balance in the body.[1]

Our modern reaction is to rush to the doctor for an antibiotic prescription or cold medicine; however, by suppressing the body's natural cleaning and detoxing process with the use of drugs, we actually damage the immune system and the electrical circuitry of the body.

In this chapter, we discuss some of the many ways we assault our immune systems electrically—many of them in the belief that we are promoting good health.

IMMUNIZATIONS

The only way the immune system builds up strength and resilience is to naturally experience the factors that will trigger its response. This process was the original logic behind immunization. However, immunization is an entirely different animal from the natural fortification process that occurs in the body. For example, when one gets a cold, the "chill" puts the immune system under stress, so that any viral activity in the body (there is some viral loading at all times in the body), takes this opportunity to have a population explosion. The "cold" is the response to this immune stress and the resulting imbalance in the microflora/ viral activity. The body uses this imbalance to trigger a "spring clean," which we experience as the cold. In essence, the cold is the body cleaning and correcting itself.

Immunization ignores this chain of events and in fact says the microorganism that the body is using to trigger its clean-up is the disease and attempts to trigger the body to attack and kill that particular microorganism. The microorganism is not the problem; it was always meant to be there. From an electrical point of view, immunization is based on an erroneous premise. Immunization is an electrical bombardment that devastates the ability of the body to control its microorganism population naturally.

Injecting the microorganism into the muscle tissue is a totally unnatural way for it to get into the body. It is impossible to produce in a laboratory that which millions of electrical interactions produce in our incredibly complex bodies. Not one of the microorganisms in a vaccination contains the same frequency or the same electrical matrix of any microorganisms already existing in the body. So how can they accurately trigger the body's defenses? In fact, these foreign substances can only be perceived by the body as poison. This is the cause of the toxic shock syndrome that sometimes accompanies immunizations.

Unfortunately, we are unwittingly allowing our children to be injected with disease-causing toxic substances that produce dramatic long-term electrical damage that can manifest as many "diseases," including malaise, fibromyalgia, multiple sclerosis, and a host of other nervous system disorders, hives, allergic asthma, anaphylaxis (a severe, potentially life-threatening allergic reaction), respiratory infections, gastrointestinal problems, eye problems, blood pressure changes, paralysis, and many other nervous and immune system malfunctions.

To inject into the tissue any potentially life-threatening and toxic substance has to run the risk of causing a toxic shock effect. In fact, vaccination is statistically known to kill 3 percent of its recipients. In a medical clinic where I work, a woman suffered a life-threatening emergency that lasted in excess of eight hours as a result of toxic shock induced by a flu vaccination given earlier at another clinic.

The germ theory of disease stems from the research of Frenchman Louis Pasteur, but the true researcher in Pasteur's institute was the eminent scientist Antoine Bechamp. Bechamp, a man without public savvy, argued all his life that disease was caused by disharmony and imbalance of the body's natural microflora; but his boss, Pasteur, who was being funded by his friends in the rapidly growing pharmaceutical industry, promoted the idea that bacteria caused disease and that bacteria could be killed by drugs. Our entire germ-based microorganism-killing pharmaceutical industry grew from this erroneous scientific premise.

On his deathbed, Pasteur apologized for deliberately taking Bechamp's research out of context so that his institute could benefit from the funding that was coming from the newly emerging drug companies. In fact, he admitted that he was wrong and that Bechamp was right. By then, however, the drug companies and their "kill-the-germs-at-all-cost" system had become entrenched; and today, our health-care system is a direct legacy of this lie. (See the original research writings of Pasteur and Bechamp, or the books *Pasteur Exposed*, by E. Hume, and *The Dream Lie of Louis Pasteur*, by R. B. Pearson, to find out more.)

Unfortunately, some schools refuse entry to children who have not been immunized. The reasoning behind this ruling is that the unimmunized children's disease-carrying potential is a threat to the remainder of the children. The logic here seems to be rather twisted. The very reason that most of the children were immunized was the belief that those children who had been immunized would no longer be susceptible to the disease. If that were so and there was an outbreak, then surely only the unimmunized children would be at risk. The immunized ones would be safe, would they not?

If any school gives immunization as a condition of entry, ask the district or governing body to supply you with a written statement that if you vaccinate your child to fulfill their entry requirements, they would take full responsibility for any "adverse vaccine reactions." No insurance company in the world will cover these—the risk is too high.

Some years back, in my search for answers to the whole immunization problem, I had the opportunity to visit a playgroup that was attended by one- to four-year-olds. I positioned myself where I was able to see the entire playground and observe the children's behavioral patterns. I ranked each child's physical vitality and speed of movement and observed their mental dexterity. After an hour's observation and subsequent note-taking, twenty-one members of the group had a relatively similar score, but the remaining three scored much higher than the main group.

At the parents' coffee break at the end of the playgroup, I approached the mothers of the three exceptionally scoring children and asked them if they had immunized their children. Each of the three mothers answered that they had not. Upon further investigation of the group, I found that they were the only three children attending who had not been immunized.

My belief, based on years of clinical experience and observation, is that the electrical bombardment from immunization can have a profound adverse effect on our health and vitality that we can sometimes carry into adulthood. If the body is able to function in perfect electrical harmony without its immune system being destroyed by incorrect nutrition, doctor- or food-induced chemical poisoning, and toxic bombardment, the strength of its own immunity is the best defense against disease states developing.

To ensure the body's perfect harmony from the beginning, breast-feeding of infants for as long as physically possible is of extreme importance. It is also highly recommended that children be kept free of chemically altered food and allowed to interface fully with soil and natural environments—permitted to crawl around in the dirt and ingest a bit of soil—so that their bodies, it is hoped, get some natural bacteria to fortify their system.

Historically, there is evidence that suggests that immunization is ineffective. Smallpox, polio, and all other diseases whose demise has been credited to immunization were in fact on the decline naturally before the start of immunization. As smallpox and polio immunization was started, the downward trend of these two diseases leveled off and actually started to go up again. In the case of polio, immunization *gave* many people the disease. If left to run its own natural course, the disease would have been at an all-time low years earlier.

According to the British Association for the Advancement of Science, childhood diseases decreased 90 percent in England between 1850 and 1940, paralleling improved sanitation and hygienic practices, well before mandatory vaccination programs. Infectious disease deaths in the United States and England declined steadily by an average of about 80 percent during this century (measles mortality declined over 97 percent) prior to vaccinations.

The Foreign Ingredients in Vaccines

Immunization shots contain viruses and bacteria that are grown in pig or horse blood, rabbit brain tissue, dog and monkey tissue, chicken and duck eggs, and calf serum. These nonhuman antigens cause electrical chaos in the human body. Foreign substances that have not been filtered through the body's normal digestive processes can be highly toxic when injected into the muscles or lymphatic and blood systems.

Some foreign additives also normally found in various vaccines include:

- Formaldehyde—a known carcinogen

- Thimerosal—an antiseptic that is 49-percent mercury

- Aluminum potassium sulfate

- Aluminum phosphate—also used in deodorants

- Lactalbumin hydrolysate

- Phenol (carbolic acid)—extremely toxic

- Acetone—volatile and can easily cross the placental barrier and enter a fetus's system

- Glycerine—an alcohol derived from decomposed fats that can damage the kidneys, liver, lungs, and local tissue (that's the cell damage at the injection site) and can cause excessive urination and possible death

Infant Immunizations

It is not without reason that in some Asian countries, where they have a greater understanding of the electrical makeup of the body, infant immunization is largely outlawed before two years of age. They know that the infant's immune system is not strong enough to handle the possible toxic effects of immunization. In most Western countries, it is required that immunization be carried out *prior* to two years of age. Disease in the Western world far exceeds that of these Asian countries.

In Japan, the raising of the minimum vaccination age to two years was followed by the virtual disappearance of crib death and infant convulsions. Under pressure from the pharmaceutical companies, the country allowed three-month-old and older babies to be vaccinated in the 1980s, and the incidence of crib death increased again.

In a study of children in kindergarten through grade 12 reported in the *New England Journal of Medicine* in 1989, 60 percent of the children vaccinated contracted the disease they were "immunized" against.[2] A large epidemic of diabetes (80-percent increase) occurred in New Zealand following a recent hepatitis B immunization program, and research scientists believe the most likely explanation is that the immunization program caused the diabetes epidemic.[3] Two-thirds of 103 children studied who died of SIDS (sudden infant death syndrome) had been vaccinated within the last three weeks, many dying within a day of vaccination.[4] When childhood vaccination rates dropped in Australia by 50 percent, SIDS also dropped by 50 percent. Following the introduction of compulsory immunization, the incidence of diphtheria *increased* by 39 percent in France and 55 percent in Hungary, it tripled in Switzerland and increased from 40,000 to 250,000 in Germany, mostly affecting immunized patients. On the other hand, in Sweden, diphtheria virtually disappeared without the need for immunization.

There is a plethora of information available about the ineffectiveness of vaccines in preventing epidemics. Measles and mumps outbreaks have occurred in vaccinated populations.[5,6] One study found that measles vaccination "produces immune suppression, which contributes to an increased susceptibility to other infections."[7] Japan experienced yearly increases in smallpox following the introduction of vaccines in 1872. By 1892, there were 29,979 deaths, and all victims had been vaccinated.[8] In the early 1900s, in the Philippines, 8 million people received 24.5 million vaccine doses and the death rate quadrupled. In 1989, Oman had a widespread polio outbreak six months after achieving complete vaccination.[9] There are many more related studies and cases,[10] but the above examples serve to show that the effectiveness of vaccinations is highly questionable.

Medically, the 3-percent death rate resulting from immunization shots falls within the "acceptable risk" category. Ask the parent who has just lost a child as a result of childhood immunizations whether this is an "acceptable risk." It is very difficult for a mother to come to terms with the death of a previously perfectly healthy baby within days, and sometimes within hours, of childhood immunization shots.

Flu Vaccinations

Each year, we are told to get the "shot" for the newest strain of flu. The problem is that the "newest strain" was the one that was injected into us last year and caused a toxic loading. In its mutated and electrically distorted form, it was able to survive in our body and mutate again. In our bodies' attempt to rid themselves of this toxin, we "caught" a cold or mild flu and then spread it around with our breath until it took hold in someone with a low immune system, mutated slightly again, multiplied, and came back to us as the "new strain." This process takes six to twelve months, hence the recommended shots every six to twelve months.

The only way to guarantee the development of even more flu strains is to keep vaccinating. What a wonderful money-making idea—never mind the continual hammering of our immune systems in the process.

The outbreak of foot-and-mouth disease (which is a bovine flu) in the United Kingdom in the early months of 2001 is an interesting example that relates directly to this discussion. At the highest levels of government, with pressure from the farmers, vaccinations for foot-and-mouth were vehemently opposed, because the farmers knew that vaccinations would perpetuate the disease and not curtail the problem. It is strange that in agriculture, vaccinations are so actively opposed; whereas in the human health field, vaccinations are strongly recommended. It makes one wonder whether the human vaccination program is about stopping a problem or about making money for the manufacturers and suppliers of the vaccinations.

A number of years ago in New Zealand, the national government, responding to information given to it from its Department of Agriculture, banned all immunizations against brucellosis (a type of flu in cows that can cause miscarriages) in the dairy and beef cows in order to finally eradicate the disease. Once again, we have agricultural science proving our point that immunization does not stop the disease but only prolongs its continued survival.

A well-known flu epidemic—the "Spanish Flu" of 1918–1919—killed a large percentage of the world's healthy population. This was largely the result of flu vaccination of American soldiers before leaving for Europe during World War I. The flu then mutated in their bodies, and they spread it throughout Europe. More young males died of the Spanish flu than were actually killed in battle. An estimated 675,000 American civilians were killed by this epidemic, 225,000 in Britain, and 6 million in India—20 million worldwide.[11] Vaccinations proved to be a deadlier weapon than anything the Germans threw at the allies.

There are many reported cases of deaths from flu soon after the administration of flu shots. Toxic shock resulting in death from "shots" is far more widespread than most people realize. The medical establishment works hard to keep the truth from becoming public knowledge.

The United States federal government's National Vaccine Injury Compensation Program (NVICP) has paid out over $1.2 billion to parents of vaccine-injured and -killed children, a rate of close to $90 million taxpayer dollars per year.[12] Insurance companies (who do the best liability studies) refuse to cover adverse vaccine reactions.

Rubella Immunizations

Among teenage girls, the greatest number of those who suffer from rubella are those who have been immunized against it. The sad thing about childhood immunization, particularly against rubella, is that it often worsens the problem from a relatively harmless childhood disease to many more severe and devastating problems later in life, including birth defects and miscarriage. As reported in *Science* magazine, in 1970 as many as 26 percent of children who received the rubella vaccination developed rheumatic fever or rheumatoid arthritis later in life, according to the Department of Health, Education, and Welfare.

Measles Vaccinations

According to the *Journal of the American Medical Association:*

> *A vast number of children who were injected with measles vaccine between 1963 and 1968 in the United States are now subject as young adults to what is called "atypical measles." This is a very severe form of the disease in which it now appears that, because of the vaccination, there is an increased susceptibility to measles viruses, resulting from a damaged immune response.*[13]

A review of sixteen hundred cases of measles in Quebec, Canada, between January and May 1989 revealed that 58 percent of the school-age cases were in children who had been previously vaccinated. This could hardly be classified as a successful endeavor! Once again, when will we learn what agriculture science has known for many years—that immunizations only maintain the disease, not eradicate it?

Meningitis Vaccinations

In 1998 there was an article in the *Vancouver Sun* about the death of a teenage girl in Ontario, Canada.[14] The article mentioned that she died of meningitis a week after she had been vaccinated against it. The article skirted around the relationship of the injection to the cause of her death. This could be considered a classic case of immunization-induced, or toxic shock, death.

Immunization in all its forms, for whatever reason, means bombing the body's immune system. It has not gone unnoticed that the destruction of the immune systems of the people of northern and central Africa has taken place since the World Health Organization went in and started mass immunization in the 1970s. In fact, the advent of AIDS (which is an immune system failure with resulting viral attack), which some claim originated in Africa, became evident only after this widespread and repeated immunization program. (For more information on this topic, read *Full Disclosure* by Dr. Gary Glum, available in HTML format by e-mailing Dr. Glum at drglum@attglobal.net.)

DRUG USE

Another of the "body bombs" that destroys the immune system function is the use of recreational drugs. Ecstasy, hashish, heroin, LSD, and other recreational drugs cause chronic circuitry damage in our electrical bodies. Drug users' bodies very seldom recover their pre–drug-use vitality, though there are exceptions, of course, due to various resilient parameters in different people. In terms of life-force energy, a hard drug user is very easy to distinguish, and even ex-users hold the damage within their energy fields for many, many years. In some ways, the body never fully recovers from hard drug use.

Often the electromagnetic energy fields around the body are so damaged that the physical body shows symptoms such as inability to concentrate, indecisiveness, lack of direction, mood swings, a greater requirement for sleep, loss of luster in the skin, slow wound healing, loss of hair tone, and sometimes the development of bulging eyes. This last symptom is a classic symptom of damage to the crown chakra, the part of the energy system at the top of the body. This is more predominant when harder, narcotic and psychedelic drugs have been used repeatedly.

The devastation to the body's energy system caused by recreational drug use is sadly often duplicated with prescription drugs. However, the rebuilding of the body is possible if the former user is prepared to invest in his or her own recovery by taking high levels of electrically available minerals, vitamins, and some very specific electrically formulated herbal combinations. For every year that one has taken drugs, the recovery to full vigor and electrical function within the body, if at all possible, would take in the vicinity of three months.

Recovery from the degeneration associated with our modern lifestyles would be one month for every year, which is the normal accepted standard within the natural health industry. This shows that to rebuild the body physically and electrically from drug use is three times more difficult than rebuilding the body from the normal traumas and stresses of daily life.

CHEMOTHERAPY

One of the biggest bombs by far that we could ever expose the body to is chemotherapy. Its effects on our electrical system could be compared to those of a string of napalm bombs detonated on a forest. Very little is left alive or functioning afterward.

The recovery rate of cancer sufferers who elect surgery and chemotherapy as treatment is frighteningly low. More money and more so-called research hours have been allotted to cancer in the last forty years with the least amount of success than for any other single ailment. Cancer is still one of the biggest killers. One would think that after more than forty years of research and treatment that has gotten us nowhere, our medical system would accept the fact that it has to look in other directions. Sadly, the opposite has been the case. Every time anybody in the world has come up with a new approach in an attempt to alleviate the horror of cancer, they have either been legislated out of existence or been belittled beyond belief.

As Linus Pauling, double Nobel Laureate, said, "Everyone should know that the 'War on Cancer' is largely a fraud." The "War on Cancer," like the "War on Crime" and the "War on Drugs," should perhaps be seen as self-perpetuating industries and *not* as attempts to find solutions that would put them out of business. One example is the Essiac fiasco that has been ongoing in Canada since the 1930s. Essiac is a combination of natural herbs long used by Northern Canadian Indians. It has the most proven track record of alleviating cancer and dramatically lowering pain associated with advanced cancer that I know of. It has no known side effects and has been used successfully by thousands of people; however, the selling and administering of this formulation as a cure for cancer is illegal. In fact, the book *Calling of an Angel*, by Dr. Gary Glum, which thoroughly documents Essiac and its cancer-reducing properties, is no longer in print in the United States; as Glum said he encountered too many problems from the federal government as a result of his publishing of the book. (See Appendix A for information on obtaining Glum's book in HTML format.)

How any politician or medical industry or pharmaceutical company shareholder can have a clear conscience over this and the deliberate suppression of many other natural treatments is almost unbelievable. The medical profession's line of attack for cancer is to load the body up with life-destroying toxic substances (chemotherapy and radiation), whereas the natural health industry works to assist the body to come alive in all areas. It is an extremely strange concept that one would use the strongest life-destroying drugs in the belief that by doing so life would be enhanced. The cancer establishment is fixated on damage control—diagnosis, treatment, and basic genetic research—and is indifferent, if not hostile, toward cancer prevention—getting carcinogens out of the environment.

Interestingly, there are significant conflicts of interests on the parts of the National Cancer Institute (NCI) and the American Cancer Society. In his book *The Politics of Cancer Revisited*, Dr. Samual Epstein goes into great detail about the conflicts of interest between the American Cancer Society and the cancer drug, mammography, pesticide, and other such industries.[15] He charges that the cancer establishment is misleading people into believing that it is spending a good chunk of its stashed-away billions on prevention, which is untrue. Looking for high crimes and misdemeanors? Read Dr. Epstein's book.

It is my belief that cancer is very preventable and recoverable, particularly in the early stages of diagnosis before surgery is required. Once surgery has been undertaken, electrical reconstruction using advanced vibrational medical knowledge is almost a requirement for the body to be able to complete the healing process. If this electrical reconstruction is not carried out, the recurrence of cancer somewhere in the body within five years is almost guaranteed. With the correct electrical work and a perfectly healthy natural diet, in cooperation with the input of megadoses of electrically available herbs, vitamins, and minerals, the recurrence of cancer is largely nonexistent.

Am I suggesting that cancer can be cured? If that means returning the body to its electrically harmonious precancerous state, my answer would be an unequivocal "Yes," based on my clinical experience. With what is known in the natural health field, particularly in vibrational medicine, and by using electrically available and formulated herbs, minerals, and enzymes in the right doses at the initial diagnosis of cancer, there is the potential to bring cancer into the extremely "curable" arena. However, if the client has elected chemotherapy bombardment, recovery and nonrecurrence are exponentially harder to achieve. A good source on this matter is *Questioning Chemotherapy* by Ralph W. Moss, Ph.D.[16] Electing to go the chemotherapy route is often the same as signing your own death warrant. The electrical reconstruction of the body's energy system using all that the natural health industry has to offer is sometimes not enough after chemotherapy. However, in my experience, the success rates are still "hundreds of percents" better than going only the "traditional medical" way.

DISHARMONIOUS ELECTROMAGNETIC FREQUENCIES (EMFs)

Even though North America is ruthless in its suppression of anything that slightly deviates from the gospel according to the drug industry, some countries are starting to wise up to electrical truths pertaining to disease.

I quote the following from a display in the Schweiz National Science Museum, in Lucerne, Switzerland:

Electromagnetic Vibration. How our cells communicate: All healthy cells in the body can receive and communicate vast amounts of information in the form of ultra fine electromagnetic vibrations. Along with vibrations in the natural environment (sunshine, for example) they shape all the body's biological processes. Techniques such as acupuncture and homeopathy have shown that a communication block between cells, rather than biochemical disorders, is often the cause of illness. From this point of view, the increasing concentration of artificial waves in the environment is bound to cause problems. Radio, radar and microwaves effectively "jam" the exchange of information between cells, and so may provoke illness.

This statement, approved by some of the world's foremost scientists for public display in a science setting of this standing, had a profound effect on me. It validates everything I have been trying to educate people about. It validates more than fifteen years of my work and the reason for this book. This scientific statement shakes the very foundation of our present medical belief structure. It is the first public scientific statement I have seen that rebuffs the decades of misinformation used by our drug-based medical system derived from the admittedly incorrect Pasteur theory. As the statement says, "vibrations shape *all* the body's biological processes."

Vibrations that the body cannot recognize as natural—those that did not evolve as part of nature—also shape the body's biological process. Toxic chemicals and pharmaceutical drugs, immunizations, manufactured food, chemical food coloring, artificial sweeteners, pesticides, and herbicides all contain unnatural vibrations. Likewise, artificial wave sources include not only radio, radar, and microwaves but also cell phones, X-rays, CT scans, ultrasound, and all other frequencies (waves) that science and our modern civilization in their wisdom have bestowed on us.

All of these disharmonious waves effectively "jam" the exchange of information between cells and *provoke* illness. As the body is an electrical being, every aspect of every function is an electrical transmission, an electrical communication. To compromise any of these electrical communications causes *disease.*

In the European Court of Human Rights on August 25, 1998, a Swiss federal court verdict against a Dr. Hans Ulrich Hertel was overturned. Dr. Hertel was originally sued because he had said that microwaves cause cancer. In an article published in the *Franz Weber Journal,* he wrote that "food prepared in microwave ovens damages health and leads to changes in the blood of consumers and said changes point to a morbid disturbance which could be the beginning of a cancerous process."[17]

The European court judgment was a severe reprimand of the Swiss court, which had unanimously and without public trial issued judgment in favor of the Swiss Association of Electroapparatuses for Household and Industry against Dr. Hertel. The European court, after calling experts from throughout the scientific community, passed judgment that the Swiss court was wrong and Dr. Hertel was right. The Swiss court then issued a proclamation that all public restaurants that use microwaves must inform their clientele, by public signage, that microwaves may be in use in that public establishment. The Swiss Health Department also issued a general health warning against the use of microwaves.

It is generally public knowledge in many European countries that microwaved food is a health hazard, and in fact the production and sale of microwave ovens in Europe is grinding to a halt. Incredibly, in the United States of America very few people seem to be aware of the risk.

That an energy communication takes place between every frequency of energy in this cosmos, and thus between human beings and each cell, is a scientific fact. "Traditional" medicine ignores this truth. But though Galileo was condemned to death for challenging the scientific truths of his day, it was nonetheless true that Earth circled the sun.

ASPARTAME

It may be evident what an electrical disaster sugar is; but sadly, common replacements for sugar, and many diet products that contain an ingredient called aspartame, are possibly even more potent poisons.

Dr. H.J. Roberts, an internist specializing in endocrinology and neurology and the author of *Aspartame: Is it Safe?* and *Defense Against Alzheimer's Disease: A Rational Blueprint for Prevention,* has looked at some of the effects of aspartame on the nervous system. According to Dr. Roberts, aspartame can aggravate or accelerate multiple sclerosis (MS), or even cause MS symptoms in those who do not have the disorder, resulting in misdiagnosis. In his practice, he has found that a number of his patients were incorrectly diagnosed as having MS on the basis of their various neurological and eye complaints and were more likely suffering from reactions to aspartame. "The frequency with which erroneous diagnosis of multiple sclerosis was made in aspartame reactors deserves special attention," Roberts said. "This is particularly true among young women who develop visual and neurological problems while consuming considerable amounts of aspartame products. In my opinion, this diagnosis ought to be deferred at least several months after abstinence from aspartame to enable sufficient observation for spontaneous recovery."[18]

Aspartame is composed of phenylalanine, aspartic acid, and methanol. According to Dr. Russell Blaylock, neurosurgeon and author of *Excitotoxins: The Taste that Kills,* aspartic acid literally stimulates the neurons of the brain to death, causing brain damage of varying degrees.[19]

Phenylalanine lowers the body's serotonin levels,[20] which can trigger such problems as manic depression, suicidal tendencies, mood swings, panic attacks, insomnia, anxiety, hallucinations, and rage.

When aspartame is heated beyond 86° F, the methanol is converted into formaldehyde and then into formic acid, which can cause, among other problems, metabolic acidosis—a disturbance of the body's acid-base balance in which the acid level is too high. At first, aspartame was used in only a few hundred products, but now it is in more than

5,000 products, including diet drinks, soda, ice cream, gum, prescription drugs, and baked goods. When the FDA approved aspartame, it didn't mention that the substance should not be heated. It should be noted that the human body operates at approximately 97° F, so even if aspartame is not used in cooked goods, when we eat or drink something containing it, the body will bring it above the danger limit and turn it into a dangerous neurotoxic substance. Perhaps the health problems experienced by the servicemen and servicewomen in Desert Storm can be linked to the consumption of soda containing aspartame that sat in the 120-degree sun for weeks at a time?

Several studies have linked aspartame consumption to brain tumor growth and grand mal seizures in lab animals.[21-25] Toxicologist Dr. Adrian Goss told a congressional hearing that aspartame caused cancer in lab animals.[26]

In 1995, the FDA documented ninety-two symptoms (or electrical malfunctions) associated with aspartame, from coma to death. Among them are headaches, dizziness or problems with balance, nausea and vomiting, abdominal pain and cramps, change in vision and other eye problems, diarrhea, seizures and convulsions, memory loss, fatigue, weakness, rash, change in sensation (numbness, tingling), oral sensory changes, menstrual changes, localized pain and tenderness, urogenital problems, swallowing difficulty, metabolic problems, speech impairment, miscellaneous gastrointestinal problems, fainting, cardiovascular problems, respiratory problems, edema, change in hearing, unspecified muscle tremors, change in body weight, change in thirst or water intake, blood glucose disorders, hallucinations, dental problems, change in smell, blood and lymphatic problems, difficulties with pregnancy, developmental retardation in children, change in breast size or tenderness, change in sexual function, shock, and death. In other words, aspartame is associated with a long list of severe adverse reactions, yet still it is allowed to proliferate our foods. Aspartame consumption could also be linked with the increase in chronic fatigue syndrome, systemic lupus, fibromyalgia, multiple sclerosis, and Alzheimer's and Parkinson's diseases. Many practitioners have noted that when patients suffering from these "diseases" stop ingesting products containing aspartame, their symptoms diminish dramatically within months. It can be noted that the increase in aspartame in our food has corresponded with a parallel increase in the above-mentioned diseases, particularly Alzheimer's and Parkinson's diseases. Aspartame is like an electrical hand grenade in the body—avoid it at all costs!

And aspartame is not even effective as a diet product. According to Mission Possible, an organization committed to educating people about the devastating effects of aspartame, the ingredient makes people crave carbohydrates, which cause weight gain! Dr. Roberts says that his patients lose an average of 19 pounds per person when he gets them off aspartame. Most of the information in this section was obtained from Mission Possible. To read the full text from Mission Possible, see www.dorway.com.

SUMMARY

As we have discussed, there are many electrical body bombs that can compromise the body's immune system and endocrine system functions, which in turn affects our health and well-being. By being aware of these body bombs and their devastating effects, we can make conscious choices of alternatives that will enhance our well-being rather than jeopardize it. In the chapters to come, we will address what you can do on a daily basis to strengthen the body's immune system and fortify your electrical circuitry. We will also offer practical suggestions on what to do to rectify the effects of these body bombs. But first, let us look at another major experience that can have a devastating long-term effect on the health and well-being of an individual—his or her entry into this world.

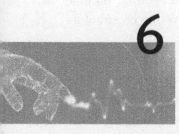

6

Birth's Electrical Traumas
and Their Remedies

I was fortunate that for the first forty years of my life I interfaced on a daily basis with animals. From my early twenties I was responsible for overseeing the births of up to 500 cows annually. If you like, I am an extremely experienced midwife.

The reproductive system of that wonderful bovine, the domestic cow, is practically identical to the human reproductive system. In fact, all of the artificial insemination, in vitro fertilization, female egg extraction, fertilization, and replanting techniques that are now used as relatively common practice in assisting women to become pregnant resulted from knowledge gained in the dairy industry.

The New Zealand dairy industry leads the world with its fertility knowledge, which is the benchmark by which medical science sets its standards. Since I lived and breathed this industry, I was very aware that to have a cow with calving difficulties usually meant that she was not able to fully lactate as quickly as one who did not, so it was extremely economically advantageous to have the cows calving naturally with the least amount of problems.

After twenty years or so of assisting in difficult births on the farm, I was able to see the difference in behavior of the mother and her young resulting from a difficult birth as compared to those with natural, trouble-free births. Many times after I have assisted with a difficult birth, the mother has subsequently totally rejected her young. Yet in a natural, unassisted birth, a mother's rejection of her young is extraordinarily rare.

This observation of cows has influenced how I have looked at some of the problems of the mothers and children who have ended up in my clinic. During my years of clinical experience, countless hundreds of children have been brought to me with symptoms ranging from asthma to spina bifida. I initially started to question each mother who brought in an ill child about their birth experience and the immediate postbirth treatment of the child. It soon became glaringly obvious that the greater the childhood disease state that had manifested, the greater the disharmony the child had suffered immediately postbirth. The mother's postbirth depression also could be traced to the disharmony experienced straight after birth.

Once I had established this physical correlation I then looked at the electrical matrix of the child's energy system to trace the physical symptom back to the electrical malfunction and then back to what caused the electrical malfunction. At this point I made a frightening discovery.

In nearly every case of childhood asthma, allergies, and many other health problems, the energy circuits that govern lung function were "blown out" as a result of doctor-induced traumatic shock. This shock, in every case, was the result of a doctor's extreme physical abuse, which was in the form of the proverbial "smack on the bottom" when the infant first came out of the womb.

How is it that doctors can physically assault an extremely sensitive young being and not be aware of the absolute horror, shock, and torment that young being must feel? Are our medical professionals so extremely naïve as to believe that a newborn child is incapable of feeling and reacting to such an extreme stimuli?

This assault would have the same effect, when one looks at the electrical damage that occurs, as an adult whose car goes out of control and goes over a hundred-foot bank, crashing down and hitting all sorts of rocks and trees on the way. The person survives the crash, but, as you can imagine, there would be serious psychological and emotional disturbances as a result of the trauma. The electrical circuitry damage would also be great and would cause many physical problems downstream. Such persons would have been terrified out of their minds, and their bodies would be in shock for days, if not weeks, after the accident.

To deliberately put a newborn infant through this degree of trauma is totally unacceptable and unnecessary in any situation. The reasoning given for this physical battering is that doctors believe it is required to start the breathing process. How, then, was every animal and every human being able to survive and start breathing since time began?

The entire modern birthing process that is carried out in most hospital situations is abusive to both mother and child. I have been called to assist many mothers in their birthing process and as a result have seen the amazing difference in the child's behavioral patterns and subsequent health, as well as the mother's emotional state, resulting from the immediate postbirth experience being traumatic or nontraumatic.

It is my experience that hospital births have a greater adverse effect on mother and child than midwife-assisted or home births. I am a passionate believer in the dehospitalization of the birth process in all ways. Giving birth is not a disease and in no way should be treated as such.

From an electrical understanding, based on the many thousands of children I have seen over the years in my clinic work, I have never found any residue trauma in the electromagnetic energy fields (aura) of the newborn as a result of the experience the fetus went through traveling the birth canal. However, during this part of the birth, the mother can sometimes experience extreme anxiety and discomfort (birth is very rarely perfectly harmonious for the mother). The fetus appears not to be traumatized by this natural process and does not appear to take any disharmonic frequencies from the mother when she is giving birth. (Please note: We are not talking about the blood transfer problems or chemical toxicity that can occur as a result of the mother's state of health; we are focusing here on the electrical aspect of the birthing process.) The experience the child has at the time of its birth is totally controlled by the human beings who are assisting at the birth. Environmental factors—hot, cold, in a house, in the back seat of a car, or out in the bush or a field—do not appear to have any adverse impact on the traumatic loading of the infant's energy fields. The only traumatic loading that occurs is as a result of the human interface between the infant and those in attendance, including the mother.

To place the mother on her back during the birthing process is to go against every way the body and nature works. Gravity pulls the baby down toward the mother's back, often resulting in lower back pain for years. To have the mother on her back may be beneficial to an attending doctor, but one would have to question why the doctor is telling the mother what should be and what should not. Who is having the baby, the doctor or the mother?

Imagine for a moment that you spent nine months in a tank of warm water, and the pressure of the water touching you was the only sensation your skin knew. Suddenly, without warning, you were extracted from that water, your life-giving umbilical cord was cut, you started to suffocate, and you were held up and twisted around and then experienced a severe impact. As you were lifted out of the water, the absence of any pressure against the skin would have made you feel as if you were expanding and about to explode. All of what you knew as your security—your life—does not now exist. You are instantly in a state of absolute terror and shock. You would not dare move a muscle. You would be shocked into absolute rigidity.

Unable to breathe, and with no oxygen coming through the cut umbilical cord, you were rapidly turning blue and dying. The "doctor" swung you upside down (another traumatic experience—gravity pulling on your head now outside the embryonic bath) and whacked you on your behind! At that point, you perceived your life as under total threat and you did the only thing possible—you screamed. The scream forced your lungs to prematurely start working, damaging the electrical circuitry. (Everybody smiles . . . except you!)

The proverbial smack on the bottom can cause downstream electrical chaos in the baby's body. In order to avoid that initial disharmony, here is what we consider a perfectly harmonious birth. In an electrically compatible birthing process, the mother would have completely free movement and would be able to make all the choices and be in control of who and what assistance she desired.

At the final stages of birth, she would have chosen to be either upright, in a squatting position, or semisitting, with her bottom and back supported on a bean bag, so that gravity would offer its maximum assistance. The mother, if she was given the environment that allowed her to feel safe and secure and in control, would possibly never elect to give birth flat on her back. In fact, she would probably have an overpowering urge to move around, to sway, and generally to allow her pelvic structure to loosen and open. She would naturally position herself so that gravity would assist the birthing process.

As the child emerges from the birth canal (in the perfect scenario), the mother would take its body with her hands cupped around each side of its chest and assist its final passage from the birth canal. Relaxing backward, onto the support of the bean bag, for example, she would draw the infant up onto her breasts. There, for a moment, with skin-to-skin contact between the infant and the mother's breast, and skin-to-skin contact between the infant's back and the mother's hot hands, both mother and child would rest.

The physical environment the child now experiences is as close as possible to the environment it has just left and knows so well. With its head buried in its mother's bosom, it is aware of the mother's heartbeat, which is so familiar. The wet and warm skin-to-skin contact is barely distinguishable from the experience of the embryonic fluids. The child feels safe and secure because it is cradled on one side by the mother's bosom and stomach and on the other side by the mother's hands, which are all but covering it.

In the perfect scenario, lying on your mother's naked bosom, with your body feeling the pressure of the skin contact, you felt safe and secure. You were not suffocating, as you were getting all of the oxygen that you required the same way you had for the previous nine months: through your umbilical cord.

Slowly, you become aware of your different environment, and as nature's impulses took over, you slowly moved your head. Your rested mother, responding to the same natural impulses, gently slid your warm, moist body over so that your mouth came in contact with her nipple.

Your electrical circuitry or, more correctly, the polarity between your top and bottom lip (the body's two most powerful circuits, or meridians—the governing and central—are connected to the top and bottom lips) connected with the electrical circuitry and polarity of your mother's nipple and the areola (the darker color skin around the nipple). The resulting electrical connection caused an instant change in your mother's hormone production. This allowed a physical stimulation in the cellular tissue of her mammary gland and an electrical interface between the sphincter muscle in the nipple and the fluid contained within the mammary gland, resulting in the physical expression of colostrum, the milk secreted shortly after giving birth.

In this scenario, the infant, having an instantaneous reaction to stimuli from the warm colostrum, acts on a natural instinct and searches for more (in fact, the natural instinct is once again a complex electrical process). As the infant's lips make repeated contact with the nipple and the areola, more colostrum flows, and the infant responds by suckling. As the infant starts to suckle and swallow, the electrical communication that is already taking place at the nipple allows the lung meridian (circuit) to fire. This electrical connection causes the cells of the diaphragm, followed by the upper lobes of the lungs, to start to expand and contract. Breathing starts slowly and naturally as the electrical impulses to the lung circuit increase.

As the infant's body responds to the intake of oxygen through its own lungs, an electrical message is sent from the infant back down its umbilical cord to the cells that connect the placenta to the inside of the mother's womb.

Contained within that electrical impulse is the message for the cells in the placenta to let go of their attachments, as oxygen is no longer required from this source. As the breathing increases, more electrical messages are sent to the placenta and greater numbers of cells are unbuttoned, until the placenta fully releases itself from the inside of the mother's womb. The electrical instructions for the releasing of the placenta came from the now suckling and breathing infant, not from the mother's body.

In some births, the electrical instructions that unbutton the placenta happen spontaneously, and the placenta comes away from the mothers' womb prior to the child beginning to suckle. This is quite normal in some cases, and it appears that suckling is not always necessary to stimulate the unbuttoning of the placenta. From my experience, this early releasing of the placenta prior to the suckling symbolizes a very quick, easy, and harmonious birth for the mother. As no two births are the same, and every mother's body reacts and behaves differently, there are no hard and fast rules. However, the point that needs emphasizing is that if the placenta is not spontaneously released by the mother's body, the umbilical cord should never be cut prior to suckling by the child. The suckling will create the electrical impulses to stimulate the placenta's release, and the child will have adequate levels of oxygen until its lung circuits are connected and functioning.

ELECTRICAL CHAOS SUFFERED BY MOTHERS AND CHILDREN

This section is included because of the large numbers of mothers and children I have seen in my clinic over the years who have suffered malfunctions that are largely avoidable. I hope that a greater understanding can be gained from this information that will benefit all families, particularly the mothers, as our society's well-being, in my opinion, is largely indexed to the health and vitality of our mothers and their offspring. To me, society and all its resources should revolve around mothers as a priority. I look forward to the day, hopefully in the not-too-distant future, when this becomes a reality.

Lung Damage Due to Birthing Trauma

The whack on the bottom that children often experience as part of the classic birth scenario, as in any situation when you are hit suddenly and unexpectedly, causes a reflex action, and the diaphragm spasms, which has the effect of taking in a quick sharp breath. This forced lung function prior to the natural circuitry connection, as mentioned earlier, causes severe damage to the lung circuitry. If this circuitry is not able to repair itself as the child grows, lung problems such as asthma are a guaranteed result. The predominance of lung cancer, even among non-smokers, could also be said to be directly related to this barbaric act.

To prematurely cut the umbilical cord, as is normal practice in most Western hospital birthing situations, stops the entire natural electrical process just described earlier from taking place. To cut the umbilical cord immediately after the infant emerges from the birth canal is to cut off its supply of oxygen and stop any electrical messaging between mother and child from taking place. The child becomes asphyxiated and subsequently immediately goes into traumatic shock (as you or I would if we were being suffocated).

Postnatal Depression

Because of the umbilical cord being prematurely cut, the infant is unable to send the electrical messaging that is required for the releasing of the placenta. The placenta is a part of the baby and not a part of the mother's body. As the cutting and clamping of the umbilical cord prematurely stops the blood flow through the placenta, the placenta immediately starts to become toxic. The mother's body recognizes this toxicity and goes into rejection mode, which forces the unbuttoning of the placenta in an extremely electrically disharmonious fashion. She then expels the placenta from her body.

This sets up the scenario for the extremely widespread and insidious problem that mothers suffer called postnatal depression. This is a severe emotional imbalance and at times a life-threatening depressed state. It is very easy to understand, when we look at the birthing process electrically, that the cutting of the cord before the placenta was unbuttoned by the infant forced the mother's body to go into rejection. This is a life-saving reaction on the part of the mother's body (if the placenta is not released quickly, severe toxemia may cause an extremely quick death for her).

The depression arises because the mother's body cannot distinguish between rejecting the placenta and rejecting the baby, since the placenta and the baby are electrically indistinguishable. By rejecting the placenta, her body is telling her that the baby has been rejected also.

The resulting rejection mode that the mother's body goes into has a severe impact on her. On one hand, she is holding and looking at her newly born infant with whom she is meant to be madly and passionately in love, and on the other hand, her body has gone into rejection. There is total electrical chaos. The mother's entire system can be blown out of harmony, leaving her in an emotionally devastated state. Nothing in her body will be functioning harmoniously, and in fact, the wonderful gift of breastfeeding can become a nightmare. This is the reason for postnatal depression and the devastating trauma and guilt that many mothers experience after birth.

With Caesarean births, mothers often have rejection problems similar to those who have natural births, which can manifest as postnatal depression. However, there is the possibility of the child suffering even more than the mother. The devastating effects on the child's electromagnetic system are amplified in C-section births due to the starvation effect the child experiences as a result of the antibiotic bomb the mother was given prior to the Caesarean. No hospital that I know of will operate without the cover of powerful, broad-spectrum antibiotics.

ANTIBIOTICS AT BIRTH

The mother's colostrum, sometimes referred to as the foremilk, contains live enzymes and bacteria that are essential to start the digestive process within the newborn baby's sterile stomach. Without this digestive process starting, the infant is totally unable to ferment any food, causing the effects of starvation.

The antibiotic shot given to the mother devastates the enzymes and microflora contained in her colostrum. When the baby suckles, it is getting a largely dead, unfermentable food. This is experienced by the infant as extreme discomfort and stomach cramping, similar to symptoms of food poisoning.

This is why a large number of babies that are delivered by Caesarean births lose weight dramatically postbirth and do not appear to want, or to be nourished from, the breast. A high proportion of these babies end up being fed formulas. Their discomfort is shown by extreme crying, and as soon as the formula milk is introduced, they settle and appear satisfied. This is because the formula milk contains some live enzymes and microflora that start the digestive process. However, formula milk is an extremely poor substitute for live colostrum and mother's milk.

Antibiotics and their chronic overuse in our normal medical system is another devastating bomb to the health of adults and children. I have dealt with literally hundreds of children struggling with their health as a result of indiscriminate antibiotic usage. It is my opinion that for a doctor to prescribe antibiotics, outside of a clearly serious infection or life-threatening situation, should be cause for dismissal as a health-care provider.

The use of even mild dosages of antibiotics by children totally devastates and kills a large percentage of the microflora contained in every part of their body. The resulting imbalance allows for a rapid unchecked population explosion of the naturally occurring candida fungus because antibiotics have no ability to kill candida. With a normal healthy bacterial population, candida is just one of hundreds of natural microflora and is therefore kept in its normal population context. The body bomb effect of antibiotics leaves this natural fungus with no checks and balances.

This candida problem can stay with the child into adulthood and is the underlying trigger for many, if not all, disharmonies and emotional problems developing in the body for years afterward and possibly also later on in life.

As the candida population goes up, its need for food increases. The predominant food sources candida requires are sugar and gluten (a constituent of grain, particularly wheat). This is why many people with high candida loadings have cravings for sugar and grain-based products. This drives their subsequent weight gain. Sugar and bread/muffin/pasta cravings are very often a definite sign that the microflora balance has become very distorted. To lower candida levels, *total* abstinence from sugar and grain intake is of paramount importance.

Candida

High candida loadings on the body's system due to an excess of antibiotics usage could be seen as the single biggest trigger in the development of all childhood disease scenarios. In fact, taken outside the childhood parameter, candida is the biggest single cause of non-life-threatening health problems in the Western world and is always the precursor for chronic fatigue. There are over 2,000 physical symptoms attributed to candida imbalances, and high candida levels are believed by an increasingly large number of researchers to be a major factor in the ever-increasing prevalence of cancer.

Candida growth explosion and subsequent massive symptomatic problems have been known to the top echelons of medical science since the mid 1950s. The medical profession has chosen to ignore the devastation to the human body that results from this imbalance because antibiotics were believed to be the panacea for the human race's ills—no doubt helped by the fact that antibiotics were the pharmaceutical industry's leading profitmakers for many years.

How, then, could the medical system own up to the fact that its most profitable product was the cause of nearly every disease that walked into clinics?

Then again, it may have been that antibiotics were recognized as the king hit. Every time you prescribed them, you knew that the body's immune system would be further compromised, the candida population would explode, and even more disease would ensue. You had a winner, a never-ending stream of sick people, made sick by the perceived cure. A perfect and very profitable business.

Even though candida and its related symptoms are becoming obvious to the highest echelons of medical science, the mindset and the momentum that the antibiotic industry has generated for itself is an extremely difficult juggernaut to slow or to have any hope of reversing.

Mothers often bring children to me who are suffering from multiple symptoms, such as chronic runny nose, repetitive earache, pasty-colored skin, chronic pimples, menstrual problems, irritability, dysfunctional behavior, learning difficulties, antisocial behavior, and just obviously looking as if they are struggling for survival. When I ask when the child was last prescribed antibiotics, the mother, more often than not, with tears in her eyes, draws the latest antibiotic prescription from her purse. Knowing full well that antibiotics only added to the disharmony and misery in the child's body, the mother in desperation was seeking another answer.

Candida and its related symptoms are easily seen by the trained eye. By looking at the energy field of the client, I can pick up and read the candida loading within minutes of meeting a client. One of the classic physical symptoms is redness around the upper and or lower eyelids. Other symptoms are food allergies, reactivities, chemical intolerances, and general inability to function in this modern world. These symptoms are always associated with the antibiotic-candida-microflora imbalance.

Many people, especially women, relate candida to a narrow group of problems such as vaginal yeast infections, but in fact, yeast infections, athlete's foot, severe itchiness of the skin, and so on, are just a few of the many hundreds of candida symptoms.

Allergies

I get a shocked, questioning look from mothers and others when I categorically state there is no such disease as an allergy. Allergies are the physical symptoms of the body's inability to correctly ferment and thus make electrically available the particular food that was ingested or the body's inability to detoxify environmental pollutants.

It is the body's reaction to the poisons or toxins that it produces or is subjected to that we call an allergy. Often it is possible to trace so-called allergic reactions—for example, dairy intolerance—back to the destruction of the gut bacteria caused by antibiotics (in young children, it can also be the result of the doctor-induced trauma mentioned earlier, blowing its system out). It is not the food product itself that is the cause of the allergy but rather the fact that the child/adult does not have the correct biological terrain or electrical function necessary to break down or digest the food.

In my clinical experience, Caesarean-birthed children have a higher incidence of allergies due to their stomach never receiving the full complement of live colostrum. Add these antibiotic scenarios to the electrical bombing of immunization shots at six weeks of age, and you could not create a better recipe for illness and disease if you tried.

REBUILDING GUT BACTERIA
AFTER ANTIBIOTICS

One of the easiest ways mothers and midwives can overcome the problem of having antiobiotic treatments at birth is to mix natural bacteria such as Latero Flora (See Appendix A for information on obtaining this product), *Acidophilus bifidus,* and other friendly flora with natural yogurt and smear it around the nipple and inside the baby's mouth at all of its initial suckling attempts.

The mother can also take up to 3 liters a day of this bacterial-laced natural yogurt for up to a week after her antibiotic shot. This will rebuild the microflora in her system and the life-giving aliveness of her breast milk. The infant's stomach, by getting some of the correct gut bacteria from the "fortified" natural yogurt, will be able to start its digestive process immediately and thereby be nourished by the mother's milk without the need for artificial milk formulas.

I have personally, in clinical situations, been able to see the dramatic positive results of this yogurt kickstart with Caesarean-birth babies. In these situations, the baby's birth weight is surpassed within three days and the newborn loves the breast. Normally, the baby is totally content and never cries. This, for Caesarean births, is relatively rare.

To deny a newborn infant nature's most potent food, by killing the colostrum's ability to ferment and by not rebuilding its "aliveness" and thereby its nourishment-giving qualities, is to my way of thinking, inexcusable.

The Powerful Effects of Colostrum

I have seen countless lambs and calves, showing next to no signs of life, so near death the only physical movement they could manage was a slow blink over deeply sunken and dry eyes, yet when given a few ounces of warm colostrum have been able to hold their heads up within minutes and voice their demands for more. In fact, I have had lambs brought into the house so cold and near death that normally I would have elected not to feed them. But within minutes of syringing colostrum into their stomachs, they have been running around the farm kitchen. That is the power of live colostrum.

For many years now, I have been advising a large number of my clients, in particular some cancer sufferers and others with severe digestive disorders and chronic degenerative diseases, to find a source of colostrum.

Colostrum is not milk and does not act like milk in the body. When we are born, our digestive systems and many other biological processes are not working—they had no need to, as we were living off our mothers' systems. The first fluid, called colostrum, that is expressed from the breast of mothers of all mammals, including humans, contains all the electrical triggers needed to start all functions and processes required by the body to function on its own.

The colostrum we recommend is collected from healthy New Zealand pasture-fed cows. The subsequent drying and processing of the colostrum dictates how effective the end product delivers this electrical messaging to the body. The Symbiotics Pro-Line of colostrum, which can be obtained from the Electrical Nutrition Professional company, is an industry-rated world best. (See Appendix A for more information.) It is dried and processed in the only purpose-built high-tech colostrum drying plant in existence by the world leader in dairy technology—New Zealand.

The advantage of using colostrum in the disease-recovery and health-promoting arenas is that nature supplies no better messaging system to every cell in the body to encourage them to function as they were designed to. It also supplies the perfect and complete food to ensure that cells have the energy and vitality to do just that. There simply is no better disease-recovery mechanism in nature, because colostrum contains the electrical information to tell every cell to work and how to do it.

Incredible effects from taking colostrum have been reported with improvements in libido, menstrual problems, emotional imbalances, psoriasis, irritable bowel syndrome, chronic fatigue, cancer, and on and on the list goes.

It was quite normal in the old days for the mother of a sick child to take that child to a neighboring farm and have the child suckle from the mother of a newborn. In those days, there was always one mother in the community who had just given birth. It was quite normal for children into their early teens to be treated with colostrum in this way.

It has always amazed me that the medical profession has never embraced the use of bovine colostrum for the treatment of many common illnesses. Colostrum (bovine or human) is the most powerful life-giver or immune system rebuilder that is known to exist on earth. In my clincal experience, the battle against cancer can be dramatically aided by adding extremely high levels of electrically available enzymes, friendly flora, and herbs with the added input of high levels of colostrum. (See Appendix A for more information on obtaining such supplements.) Dr. Bernard Jensen was a great example of a man who battled with cancer and won, using many of the electrically available enzymes, flora, and herbs we discussed. See his book *Come Alive* (Bernard Jensen Intl).

Colostrum can be mixed in with baby formula to supply the necessary colostrum components that are not contained in formula and that may also be missing from the mother's breast milk due to antibiotic coverage during the birthing process.

It is encouraging that some sectors of the scientific community are catching up to what natural health practitioners have been saying about colostrum for years.

The B.O.D. Strain of Bifidus

The B.O.D. strain of bifidus (B.O.D. are the initials of the agriculturist who discovered this strain) is a unique and very different natural bacterium and is one of only a few natural products that is truly effective in reducing the candida loading so prevalent in the world. In order to rebalance the microflora in the system, it is necessary to reintroduce the natural bacteria. Many natural health consultants have been recommending acidophilus for this purpose. However, although this is beneficial, on its own it will not create the balance that is required. Acidophilus bacteria does not act as a strong enough pathogen fighter and thereby does not reduce the candida count sufficiently. On its own it simply will not do the job.

With the latest scientific understanding and knowledge about stomach bacteria, we can now use the newly found natural bacteria such as the B.O.D. strain of bifidus or other electrically available flora such as *L. salivatus* and *L. plantarium* as contained in Digestive Flora, available from Avena Originals or Electrical Nutrition Professional Company. (See Appendix A for more information about obtaining these products.)

When these bacteria are combined with acidophilus, the needed decrease in the candida loading is in most cases guaranteed. In fact, using these bacteria along with adhering to a strict eating regime that eliminates all sugar and all grain is *the* most effective anticandida program. (It is suggested that you take the B.O.D. strain of bifidus and the *L. salivarius / L. plantarium* combination at different times throughout the day to maximize their potential.) The combination appears to enhance the qualities of each and is extremely powerful.

SUMMARY

A tremendous amount of knowledge is available from the natural health industry to assist mothers and children. It appears from my experience that the traditional medical system has failed miserably in its ability to understand and correct non-life-threatening but nonetheless serious, life-disrupting problems suffered by mothers and particularly their children. The natural health industry has a far greater understanding and an obvious ability to steer the young bodies back to health. There are many modalities, many components of the supplement industry and knowledge from herbology, that are very effective for most childhood problems. Traditional medicine certainly has its place in mothers' and children's health care, however, the natural health industry is, I believe, more open and willing and can assist with these kinds of problems to a greater extent. Read on to learn about more assaults on the body's electrical systems.

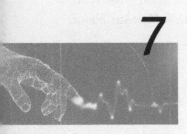

7

Downstream Effects of Electrical Body Bombs

When the body experiences ongoing bombardment from various factors that compromise its electrical system, it starts to manifest physical symptoms. These symptoms are then labeled by the medical profession and are suppressed with the help of prescription drugs. The original electrical short circuit goes unrepaired, so the body just keeps getting increasingly unhealthy. Some of the downstream health issues stem from grain toxicity and incorrect fermentation and food combining. Other malfunctions are due to the bombardment of immunizations. The ingestion of chemicals or simply the birthing process may also disrupt the electrical circuitry of the body. In this chapter, we will outline some of the common health problems that may result from the assaults to the electrical system mentioned in the previous chapters.

OBESITY

One of the main health problems resulting from grain toxicity is obesity. Obesity is now considered a severe health risk in America, according to the *Journal of the American Medical Association*. A November 1999 issue of *Time* magazine notes that more than half of all Americans are overweight.[2]

Americans have the most "fat-free" foods of any country, yet they have the highest level of obesity in the world—go figure! When I look down any busy American street, I see most people in various stages of obesity and degeneration. When I go into the malls, I see childhood obesity everywhere. As I travel in my work from Australasia to North America to Europe, it is quite obvious that the obesity and disease levels in North America are by far the highest.

I once sat down in the food court of a large mall and observed the busiest part of it, which was the place that was selling predominantly grain-based products such as doughnuts, cinnamon buns, muffins, and so on. Likewise, using the same observation technique, the most frequented aisles in the supermarket were those with the ready-made pasta and bread on the shelves. The ingestion of wheat in all its forms in North America far surpasses the nutritional requirements for carbohydrates.

When farmers want to fatten up cattle or hogs, they increase the animals' grain ration. The animals respond instantly and gain weight directly in proportion to their grain intake. But when farmers want milking cows to be lean, fit, and able to conceive every year and produce gallons of milk per day (an energy requirement), they lower the grain and increase the protein in the animals' diet. An old farm saying is "Protein for production, grain for gain."

The equation is simple: If you want to slow your body down, make it heavy, and gain weight, then ingest a high-grain diet: eat lots of wheat and other grain products like bread, hamburger buns, doughnuts, pasta and cereals. If you want to be full of vitality with lots of get up and go, with good muscle definition—that is, be lean and fit, then have a high-protein diet. These basic nutritional facts have been known in agriculture for years, yet still do not seem to be understood by many nutritionists.

LETHARGY

From an energy perspective, digestion can use up to 80 percent of the body's internal energy. We know that grains require the most energy for digestion because nature designed them not to rot, so eating a hearty muesli or cereal breakfast in the morning will give you exactly the opposite of what you thought you were going to achieve. Rather than gaining lots of energy for movement or brain power, your body will want to shut down systems in order to supply the required energy for digestion.

Remember how you felt after your last big holiday dinner—all you wanted to do was sleep. This was because digestion has priority over all other body functions. Without digestion taking place, you would die, so the body shuts down all unnecessary functions in order to have enough energy available to digest the food. In extreme cases, as after a big dinner, this process dramatically diminishes our ability to stay awake. That feeling of sleepiness takes over because your body has enforced a shutdown as a life-saving act.

With children, the body can react to stomach overload and fermentation shutdown by quickly emptying its contents (vomiting). This often happens at childrens' parties, where they tend to mostly eat grain-based foods containing sugar and to mix many different types of food (poor food combining). The children initially become extremely hyper and then their energy crashes and they get irritable and tired.

The concept of the importance of a hearty breakfast is, in fact, a carry-over from old English times. In the days of the landed gentry, the working classes had to work all day, and as payment were given one of the hunted rabbits or pheasants or a bag of grain to take home to the farm cottage to be made into the main meal of the day for the family. The lords of the manor, on the other hand, did not have to work a day for their food, and as a mark of their class, they had their main meal in the morning. The hearty breakfast originated as a status symbol and had nothing to do with good nutritional concepts.

If you want to have lots of energy and to be able to move, think, and be active in the morning, have a piece of raw fresh fruit to get you going. Fruit is more immediately available as an energy source without starting up the energy-hungry digestive process needed for grains.

Years ago when I was a dairy farmer, after milking 500 cows in the morning, my normal routine was to eat a "hearty breakfast." And what a breakfast it was: porridge with a half cup of sugar and a cup of real cream on it, followed by bacon, eggs, hash browns and toast, all washed down with a cup of coffee with milk. Upon finishing this incredible feast, my body would shut down so quickly to ensure enough energy for digestion that I would fall asleep at the breakfast table.

After learning about how the body worked, my family and I were inspired to change our eating habits. Rising at five o'clock in the morning to milk the cows, I would take with me one banana and usually two other pieces of juicy fruit and work nonstop until lunchtime and often beyond into midafternoon. My work output, my vitality, and my waistline all improved dramatically. However, I must point out that for the first two weeks or so of this change in my morning eating habit, my stomach thought somebody had cut my throat. I have never gone back to starting my day with a big breakfast since (though every now and then I have a "pig-out" day and become a couch potato, just to remind myself how good it tastes—and how bad it feels . . . I'm human!).

JOINT DEGENERATION

Another problem associated with grain toxicity and the electrical stress that results is joint degeneration, which is directly related to high wheat and grain consumption. This is a fact that has been known to agricultural science for more than fifty years. In the dairy industry, an excess of grain in the feed will give cows hotfoot—extremely tender and swollen leg joints. In horses, too much grain in the diet can lead to a symptom called foundering (or laminitis)—increased pulse rate, heat, pain, and inflammation, especially in the hoofs and joints.

In human beings, wheat or grain toxicity takes a little longer to manifest because our bodies are so amazingly evolved that they convert any excess carbohydrate into cellulite (fat) and put it away for the next famine. And we all know where that fat is. After a number of years of attempting to deal with this excess grain intake, the body's electrical circuitry starts to fail, and we feel this in the joints. If you want to guarantee joint degeneration problems from middle age on, eat a lot of grain-based foods.

In my clinical experience, I have seen arthritic symptoms—tender, swollen, and painful joints—successfully alleviated when clients have eliminated all grain and sugar from their diet and increased their protein intake. In my clinical observation, I have found that by adding an electrically formulated herbal bowel cleanse and high-quality enzymes to the client's nutritional program, the symptoms of grain toxicity can be greatly reduced.

In my opinion, the overconsumption of grain in North America is largely responsible for the prevalence of chronic obesity, lethargy, joint degeneration, and adult-onset diabetes. Furthermore, when we combine this high grain intake with sugar, this is electrically devastating and dramatically slows down cell function and can lead to extreme emotional imbalances in young children and teenagers.

DIABETES

One of the most prevalent disorders, which I believe is 100-percent induced by excess grain intake, is the "disease" commonly referred to as adult-onset diabetes. This so-called disease, in my clinical experience, often has more than a 95-percent reversal when the clients take all of the grain out of their diet for a period of at least six months. Most of my clients never go back to grain after that because they realize how devastating it was to their body and how yucky and heavy they feel when they do eat it. By grain, we mean all bread, pasta, donuts, pizza, cereals, and cookies—anything that has been made from any grain, particularly wheat, which is the worst offender.

The Mission Possible report on aspartame (an ingredient found in most sugar-free foods eaten by those with diabetes) says that aspartame is disastrous for diabetic patients even though it is recommended by the American Diabetic Association.

Diabetic patients can develop diabetic retinopathy. Many physicians do not realize that the methanol (wood alcohol, which blinded and killed skid row drunks during prohibition) in aspartame converts to formaldehyde in the retina of the eye and that this is why so many diabetics bleed and have retinal detachments. Formaldehyde is grouped in the same class of drugs as cyanide and arsenic—deadly poisons!

ATTENTION DEFICIT DISORDER (ADD)

Childhood hyperactivity and the associated problem often referred to as attention deficit disorder (ADD) are symptoms of an endocrine system overload and the resulting hormonal imbalances caused by an excess of grain-based foods, incorrect food combining, and an overabundance of sugar, artificial sweeteners, and foods containing aspartame, preservatives, and other chemicals.

It makes me extremely concerned in my clinical work when a parent brings me a young child who has been prescribed a designer drug such as Prozac. Hyperactivity and ADD are usually the "diseases" the drug treatment is being used for. The child, by this stage, often seems like a zombie, with no light in the eyes and no vigor. One mother said, "She is now very stable." I reminded her that dead is also *very* stable!

If you watch a young lamb running around the field full of life and vigor, you'll notice that it rarely does the same thing for more than two seconds at a time. One minute it will be peacefully resting. The next second it will be up and bounding around the field, jumping joyously in the air. The next second it will be racing at full speed toward its mother, nearly knocking her off her feet, for a two-second suckle at the nipple, then off again at full speed in a totally different direction. This is natural young life.

Our grandmothers reacted to this similar normal childhood behavior with: "Out of the house, you kids! Get out from under my feet and go and play somewhere else." The kids would leave the confines of the home and disappear in all directions on the farm, playing in the water puddles, building huts, playing hide-and-seek, and generally just burning up their natural, youthful vitality.

Today the child is more likely to be locked in a one- or two-bedroom apartment, with limited outside playing areas—or if there is one, it is unsafe without continual parental supervision. With this extremely limited opportunity to burn up their exuberant energy, amplified and distorted by the high levels of grain, sugar, and soda pop in their diets, in their desperate attempt to be the natural young beings that they are, their seemingly excessive behavior gets labeled as dysfunctional or hyper. Peace and quiet is not a natural behavioral pattern for the young lamb or the young child.

To force the child to fit the adult parameters of what is normal, the child is all too often given life-suppressing drugs. It is incredible that our society has lost so much knowledge of what it is to be a healthy, energy-filled child, and that we too often attempt to drug the life force from our children.

EMOTIONAL PROBLEMS

Drawing on my agricultural experience, in relation to emotional imbalances induced by grain toxicity, I will share with you some information every racehorse owner is very aware of that may be food for thought when we look at the problem behavior patterns so evident in the teenagers of North America. To make a racehorse run extremely fast with the objective of winning a race, the stable manager will slowly increase the grain ration of the horse's diet, with the intention of tweaking the horse's emotional state. This tweaking of the racehorse's emotions is intended to activate the "fight-or-flight" response (which is a slightly emotionally imbalanced state) so that when the gates open, the horse technically is slightly crazy and runs faster than normally would be possible. At times, the grain ratio is too high and the horse is so emotionally unstable that it goes crazy in the stalls before the gates are opened or runs so fast that a condition called "broken down" occurs. The result of this "breakdown" can mean that the horses' bones literally blow apart in its leg joints, and in extreme cases its heart can hemorrhage. This breakdown usually results in the animal having to be put down. In cows, excessive grain intake leads to joint degeneration, as mentioned earlier, and can make cows very "flighty."

All of these emotional and physical conditions can also manifest in human beings. Many people who eat a high-grain diet seem to be on edge all the time, very hyper, and unstable emotionally. For the type of person whose body does not convert the grain to cellulite, the high-grain diet will have a greater detrimental effect on their emotional balance and produce a very oversensitive, wired personality. This overdose of grain can lead to an emotional or mental breakdown, insanity, and chronic fatigue, to name just a few. These types of personalities in adults often succumb to alcohol dependency in order to mask their emotional imbalances.

I also believe that a large percentage of the extreme emotional instability of teenagers in our society is toxic food–based and that as a society we need to seriously look at this high-grain diet–induced problem.

ELECTRICAL MALFUNCTIONS DUE TO IMPROPER FERMENTATION

With long-term overeating and incorrect food combining (mixing crude carbohydrates and proteins), the natural electrical defenses of the cells that make up the stomach and intestinal linings start to break down. They then become physically damaged, allowing other decaying matter to seep through the porous lining of the intestinal tract into the bloodstream. This is sometimes referred to as leaky gut syndrome, but in essence an electrical malfunction is occurring. The results can include low-level blood toxicity, low energy levels, hormone imbalances, acne, emotional instability, joint pain, cellulite production (weight gain), and many other problems in the future.

Furthermore, the damage to the electrical and physical function of the cells in the walls of the intestinal tract can manifest as the disease we call ulcers. As already mentioned in Chapter 2, improper fermentation creates very sticky molecules whose behavior can lead to blocked arteries and angina smptoms and arthritis and other joint degeneration problems. In my clinical experience, taking all the grain out of the diet, separating the crude proteins and carbohydrates, and having a high protein intake has had a dramatic effect of lowering cholesterol and alleviating joint problems in many thousands of my clients. Additional problems can include kidney stones and brain-related problems like failures of short-term memory, loss of cohesiveness, balance problems, and other "aging problems." In extreme cases, major degenerative diseases like Alzheimer's disease and other motor neuron symptoms can develop.

As mentioned earlier, Dr. H.J. Roberts believes that the increase in products containing aspartame could be a major contributing factor in the escalating level of Alzheimer's disease. Alzheimer's has also been linked with the consumption of soy. A major study on the health of long-term tofu eaters, undertaken in Japan with 3,500 participants and completed in 1998, showed that tofu eaters were reported to have far more health problems than the control group. Overwhelmingly, it found the onset of serious degenerative diseases much earlier in life in the tofu-eating group, Alzheimer's being one of the main problems. This trial brought to the attention of the health authorities that the incidence of Alzheimer's in tofu eaters was the highest of any group in Japan. This trial supports the electrical nutrition concept that any food that does not contain nature's electrical matrix will cause serious degenerative problems, sooner rather than later.

OTHER PROBLEMS ASSOCIATED WITH DIET-BASED TOXICITY

We will now discuss some of the more well-known disease states that can result from our modern Western diet, which consists predominantly of toxic and dead food.

Cancer

As mentioned in Chapter 2, the slow destruction of the electrical function of the cells often leads to the cells' inability to electrically interface with its DNA code. The DNA code contains all of the information necessary for perfect physical and electrical function. By compromising the electrical interface with the DNA, the cells in essence lose contact with their instruction manual and can (and often do) manifest later in life as the disease we call cancer.

If we look at the increase in cancers of all types over the last thirty years, we see that its increase has parallels with the increase in preserved, chemically altered and chemical-laced manufactured food, immunizations, and pharmaceutical drugs.

The death rate from cancer has never been lowered by medical intervention, pharmaceuticals, or radiation. As Dr. James Compton Burnett of the United Kingdom said, "Cutting off the apples does not keep the apple-tree from growing apples." If the medical profession will not tell us the truth, then surely it is about time we used our own God-given brains and common sense.

Cancer is not something we "catch." It could be said that cancer is in fact self induced. Electrically, cancer is a massive electrical malfunction caused by a toxic and/or chemical overload that comes from the food we voluntarily eat. In the long-term preventative scenario, the only possibility for alleviating the cause is for us all to refrain from feeding ourselves and our loved ones anything that does not contain nature's electrical matrix. That would mean no sugar, nothing with artificial coloring, artificial sweetener, or preservatives, and nothing that has in any way has been changed from the way nature intended. In other words, anything out of a packet or tin or that has been processed will contain within it an electrical matrix that has the potential to cause the electrical malfunction within the body that can manifest as the disease we call cancer.

(Another electrical bombardment that adds to the risk of cancer is holding on to our emotional issues, allowing ourselves to be emotionally tight, holding on to a lot of judgments, blaming everything on everybody else, and thinking the world has given us a bad turn.)

The medical profession will never make inroads toward alleviating cancer unless it is prepared to look at the electrical damage that is the real cause. Multinational drug companies invest a lot of money in gaining the favor of doctors—hosting elaborate functions with gifts and grants for medical students and graduates, as well as the billions of dollars granted to medical teaching institutes. The multinational drug corporations have a vested interest in the cancer industry, and perhaps one could say that cancer is too good of a business to be cured. Nearly 60 cents in every medical dollar gets spent on our existing cancer scenario.

The rise in cancer rates in people also seems to correspond to the increase in cancer in our pets. Thirty years ago, working farm dogs were fed a diet of 100-percent meat, and to have a sick dog, particularly one with cancer, was unheard of. Today, however, the average farmer often feeds his dogs "hard food," which is a grain-based dog biscuit. Digestive and bowel disorders and other diseases in working dogs are now rampant, and cancer is increasingly prevalent. This is also the case in a large percentage of domestic cats and dogs that are fed large amounts of grain in their packaged hard food. When you feed a carnivore (cats and dogs) an herbivore's diet, you will eventually kill it with degenerative diseases.

As England found out, when you feed herbivores a carnivore diet, you inevitably cause total electrical chaos in the body. The cows (herbivores) were fed ground-up flesh (a carnivore's food) mixed in with their rations to increase the protein ratio so that they would produce more milk. The cows suffered a massive electrical blowout, now called mad cow disease.

We are protein eaters, we never were vegetarians (herbivores), we evolved for millions of years as hunters, we were never, before now, farmers growing and eating hundreds of tons of indigestible grain. To feed us an herbivore's diet will cause downstream electrical chaos in our bodies.

ASPARTAME POISONING

The human body operates at approximately 97° F, so when we drink our nice cool can of diet soda, it soon heats up to past the 86° F point where the formaldehyde is released from the aspartame contained in it, or any other food containing this chemical. The perfect brain neuron destruction scenario—is it any wonder our children are exhibiting symptoms of emotional problems in ever greater numbers?

SUMMARY

Electrical body bombs are creating a large portion of all the illnesses we develop in our lives, many of which have been outlined here. The only way we will be able to increase our health and vitality is to remove the causes of our electrical malfunctions and stop treating the symptoms of these body bombs instead of stopping the bombing.

Due to the widespread damage to our electrical systems, our immune systems have been continually under stress since childhood, and as we progress through our life, our immune systems are never able to attain its full, correct function. The priority in rebuilding our health and vigor would be to rebuild immune function and microfloral balance. This rebuilding process can be done with correctly formulated and electrically available natural bacteria, enzymes, minerals and herbal supplementation, which are discussed in detail in the following chapter.

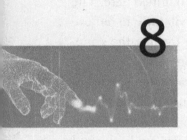

8

Remedies to Electrical Malfunctions

The first question many people ask is "Why do I have to clean up my body?" The short answer is: Because we spend a lifetime gunking it up! Our modern food intake, particularly of those foods that contain high levels of wheat and sugar, combined with our sedentary lifestyle, has the effect of slowing the body's natural cleaning systems.

Obviously, the best way of cleaning the body is to stop pouring in the electrically distorted food so that our systems might actually catch up in the cleaning departments. However, that would be an extremely slow process, and most of us would be dead as the result of the degeneration brought on by the level of toxic gunk within our system before that cleaning process was finished.

Many people are in such denial about the causes of their physical problems that they find it difficult to accept that a large percentage of everything that is going wrong in their bodies is the result of what has passed between their two lips. It has been said many times that you are what you eat. There has probably never been a more truthful statement.

The biggest difficulty we all face is that in most instances we do not believe that eating the "average" diet could cause any long-term damage. I hope that you are now starting to realize that we may be prematurely killing ourselves. Our previously held beliefs regarding food were based on completely erroneous premises and concepts.

The starting point for remedying the wrongs done to our bodies is to make raw fresh fruit and vegetables a large percentage of our food intake, accompanied by a far greater amount of crude protein than what we have been led to believe is required, and to greatly reduce our intake of grain and starches. To assist the body in all of its processes, we may combine vegetables with crude protein or with carbohydrates, but we should never combine proteins with the carbohydrates in the same meal.

The benefits of good food combining are extremely noticeable, if you make yourself aware of how you feel and your subsequent energy levels when you change your diet. The heaviness and bloated feelings after a hearty meal do not exist with correct food combinations, which suggests that the fermentation process is taking place within its correct parameters and you are not adding to the toxic loading of your system.

ELECTRICALLY ALIVE WATER

Now that we are not pouring the gunk in the top, we need to break loose the toxic buildup that is in the lower digestive tract and bowel. There are many ways that we can approach this; the best being to supplement our diet with electrically combined herbal formulations. However, without adequate levels of hydration, the process will be slow.

Water that can electrically interface with our cells is the biggest single requirement for this job. There is not one part of the body's system that can function in the absence of electrically alive water. The entire electrical function of every cellular process in the body depends on the electrical conductivity of every molecule. This conductivity increases and decreases depending on the hydration levels of the cellular structure.

We have been told that drinking water will increase the hydration of every cell within three minutes, but sadly, this is not the case. The chlorinated water we drink in today's cities and towns, even if it is filtered, cannot adequately hydrate our cells. Filtration takes out the dangerous toxic chemicals that the city council put in, but the water is still left electrically damaged or electrically dead.

This lack of hydration happens because the surface tension of this water, as a result of chlorination, which bonds the molecules of the water tightly together, is far greater than the surface tension of the body fluids that surround every cell. Even if the chlorine is filtered out, the surface tension of the water does not revert back to its natural state. The electrical bonding of the molecules of our electrically damaged drinking water is such that the water is unable to electrically interface with our body fluids. It is interesting to note that in Switzerland most of the regions and villages have made it illegal to chlorinate any city drinking or bathing water, including public swimming pools. In the United States, it is generally required that public water supplies and swimming pools be chlorinated.

The high molecular bonding and surface tension of most water is the reason why when we drink a glass of water, we have to run to the bathroom within a very short space of time. Our body's elimination system was forced to immediately dump the water, which was unable to enter our body fluids. The water, in essence, was toxic to us because of its electrical incompatibility and, therefore, could not be used to clean and flush our body tissues. Hence, the difficulty for many of us to detoxify our bodies effectively and control obesity, not to mention the extreme stress we have put our kidneys under.

This hydration issue was not a problem 100 years ago when we drank the live water nature supplied us. However, since we have moved away from the use of streams, springs, and wells, we have been forced to use chemical-laced water that even with filtration is so electrically damaged that it is largely unavailable to us. This water could be termed electrically "dead."

As a result of a lifetime of research, Doctors Patrick and the late Gael Flanagan discovered a very simple and cost-effective technique that reduces the surface tension of water to make it electrically available, the way nature had originally supplied it to us, so that it can actually be absorbed into our body fluids. Called "Microcluster technology," it is available in capsule form in a product called Microhydrin. By lowering water's surface tension, Microhydrin not only makes it more electrically available to our body fluids, but also changes its electrical conductivity potential. Microhydrin also acts as a powerful antioxidant and oxygenator of the blood. The scientific breakthrough by the Flanagans is one of the greatest advancements in natural health in decades. We can now clean the body and rehydrate it to levels previously unknown in our modern times. (See Appendix A for information on obtaining Microhydrin and another water oxygenator called Cell Food.)

There are very few (if any) other products or processes capable of achieving this because their electrical matrix will not allow that rapid interface with the cells. First, the body has to separate the electrical matrix of the H_2O molecule from the different components in the beverage before it is available for hydration. Your can of soda, your cup of coffee, or even your glass of orange juice does not do the job. There are three rules to effective hydration. The first one is alive, electrically available water. The second one is alive, electrically available water. And the third one is—you got it—alive, electrically available water.

With large numbers of people in our Western society making their livings by sitting in offices and using their brains, hydration is exceedingly important because the brain contains a greater electrical complexity than any other group of cells in the body. The only way the electrical body can function at a cellular level is through the conductivity of the fluids in and around the cells. Therefore, the hydration of the brain cells is the biggest single factor in attaining maximum brain function. Very often, people who work with their brains could alleviate the tired and fatigued feelings just by increasing their intake of electrically alive water.

Working the body physically hard is usually accompanied by heavier breathing. This increase in breathing will trigger the thirst alarm by drying the breath channels, including the mouth, and very soon you will relate this to needing another drink. However, in mental work, the trigger that we call thirst often does not fire because the increase in breathing, normally accompanying an increase in physical work, does not occur.

Our change to a nonmoving lifestyle has been faster than the body's ability to adapt and provide us with another thirst signal. As hydration levels go down, so does our electrical function. We have to be consciously aware of this lack of physical stimulation for water and be disciplined to take regular drinks throughout the course of the day. To achieve adequate hydration for maximum brain function, we would require a minimum of 1 to 1½ liters of chemical-free, electrically alive water, taken over six to eight hours.

To those people who embark on serious detoxification programs, the water intake required over a twenty-four-hour period would be up to a half gallon of water, the way nature made it—electrically alive.

Some of the symptoms of dehydration that we experience in our sedentary lifestyles are headaches; sleepiness; inability to concentrate; irritability; muscle tightness; constipation; acne; heavy, watery eyes; and general lethargy.

If you are sitting at your computer and become aware of any of these symptoms, get up, have a two-minute brisk walk around the office, and drink two or three good glassfuls of electrically available water. Most likely you will feel alive again, and your work output will jump.

LYMPHATIC DRAINAGE

More free movement, such as dance and childhood physical playing activities, is highly recommended. Gym-based workouts are designed predominantly to increase muscle strength and definition, which technically involves stripping the muscle tissue of cells. The body then replaces the lost cells with new ones, overcompensating for the damage done. This leads to the building of muscle mass. If this process is done too quickly, muscle cramping can result due to a lactic acid buildup.

The movement that is required for a detoxification process is the kind that drives the lymphatic pump without causing cell strip-down.

The lymphatic drainage system is a series of complex interrelated one-way valves called lymph nodes. These valves govern the flow of lymphatic fluid, which flows upward from the feet toward the neck, then through the subclavicle valve, which returns the lymphatic fluid to the blood for cleaning and the elimination of toxins by the liver and kidneys.

From the head, the lymphatic fluid drains down toward the neck. That is why the brain works best when we are upright, because gravity is taking care of the cell-cleaning process. But the rest of our body needs to move downward in order to drive the lymphatic fluid upward against gravity. This necessitates regular and repetitive vigorous up-and-down movements of the body as in such activities as lymphacizing, brisk walking, dancing, or even the popular exercise form TaeBo.

Most people do not realize that one of the only ways to reduce that unsightly cellulite on women and those extra inches of flab on the bellies of us men is to move it out through the lymphatic drainage system. The other way to get it out is to self-induce a famine, or, to it put plainly, starve yourself.

The only trouble with the latter approach, often referred to as fasting, is that once food intake is recommenced, the body naturally responds by increasing its efficiency of food conversion—a natural biological response. Consequently, lost cells are replaced incredibly quickly, which is why fasting achieves very little. Fasting also puts extreme stress on various systems within the body, resulting in electrical system damage, which can lead to disease. Looking at fasting from an electrical perspective, it becomes clear that there are far more effective ways of detoxifying.

Lymphacizing

Happy, joyous movement is by far the best "exercise." Free dance is definitely near the top of the list. Good brisk walking is also extremely beneficial. Lymphacizing (bouncing on an electrically tuned mini-trampoline) is the best detoxifying lymphatic draining and immune system–enhancing movement one can undertake. There are many minitrampolines on the market, but I know of only one that has been electrically tuned to the electromagnetic frequency of the body's electrical system. This electrically tuned rebounder is available in North America through Avena Originals and Electrical Nutrition Professionals. (See Appendix A for more information.) This piece of health equipment has been designed so that the frequency it produces does not damage the body's energy system, as is the case in most commercially produced minitrampolines.

With an electrically tuned rebounder, the frequency that is generated as a result of the bounce produces a vortex of energy that is compatible with the body's electromagnetic energy field. The bounce generates a field of energy because the nylon mat and the springs are being tensioned and then released. This "stress" of the mat and the springs changes the frequency within the molecules, which relates to a force field of energy being generated. On a rebounder, this energy field, or force field, is vortexed, or spun, by the outer metal band, and its amperage can be up to a thousand times stronger than the human energy field. When this generated field of energy (vortex) is out of phase with the body's energy field, the result is a yucky feeling at best and an electrical distortion in the body's fields at worst. This is why many commercially available rebounders do not feel good, regardless of the salesman's blurb.

A group of lymphologists back in the 1980s recognized this potential problem, and many thousands of dollars were spent in the scientific research and recording of the frequencies of different springs, ratios, and materials. Over a five-year period, a very sophisticated electrically tuned rebounder was developed. The rebounder we refer to is the only one in the world that we know of that has had this scientific research and tuning done to it. To the naked eye, it may look just like all the others, but just as the Model-A Ford and the newest Ferrari both have four wheels, an engine, and brakes, one has had a lot more technology and tuning, and they do the job very, very differently. An electrically tuned rebounder is a very different machine from the commonly available rebounders and will not distort the body's energy fields in any way; in fact, you will feel totally invigorated and powered up from even two or three minutes bouncing upon it. The technology actually does work. This electrically tuned rebounder is probably the most important and profound health apparatus that any of us can use.

The next most beneficial lymphatic drainage movement is brisk, arm-swinging walking. Jogging, however, actually produces about the same amount of toxins as the up-and-down movement is removing. It has been said that jogging without the shock would be the best exercise on earth. Lymphacizing (using specific bouncing techniques on an electrically tuned rebounder) does just this.

Any other exercise that requires more effort than jogging usually hinders rather than helps spring cleaning efforts. Usually such exercises produce more muscle mass and strength but do not necessarily enhance endurance, and endurance is the only indicator of fitness. Endurance is also an indication of lymphatic system efficiency. Think about this the next time you are about to rush off to the gym. Nonetheless, going to the gym is certainly better than not doing anything.

Dancing

If you do not have an electrically tuned rebounder or a gym membership and do not really want to go for a good brisk walk in below-freezing or above-melting temperatures, then how about putting on your favorite music and some comfortable clothing and literally dancing your butt off?

TaeBo is another great alternative. This is a total body workout with a large lymphatic drainage component built into it (which is quite unique in the exercise programs currently available). It blends your own hidden strength with the arts of self-defense, dance, and boxing. This incredibly popular form of exercise has spread across seventy countries. (See the resources section for information on obtaining a TaeBo videotape.)

If you spent the same amount of time per day vigorously dancing or engaging in TaeBo as is generally recommended to spend in a gymnasium, I guarantee you will achieve a greater degree of lymphatic drainage and health improvement by doing so. In fact, these activities in your own home require only your will to do it—no fancy leotards, no memberships, no fees, and no driving your polluting car to the gym. However, it is often easier to be disciplined to engage in these activities with some friends. So instead of the morning coffee meetings on your street or after-work drinks in the bar, how about a daily dance or TaeBo gathering? You will be a lot healthier and a whole lot happier.

The Problem with Bras

Do not forget, ladies, that your lymphatic drainage system has to move all the lymphatic fluid up through the lymph nodes that are contained in the outer connective tissue around your chest, including many in the mammary glands. To wear bras every waking moment goes against everything your body is trying to do to detoxify.

Wearing your bra, which is, in essence a rubber band around your chest, stops your body's cleaning mechanism. A large number of the lymph nodes, which can be referred to as chemical detox plants, are contained in your breasts, so by putting a rubber band around your chest, you are stopping the flow of fluid through these chemical detox plants. As you can see, over time, they will get congested, toxic, and polluted. To look at it another way, the exhaust pipes of your car take away the toxic waste that results from burning fuel; if you forced a potato up the exhaust pipe, your cars' engine would not function very well. The wearing of bras has the same effect as the potato in the exhaust pipe of your car.

I am not suggesting that you burn your bras, but please, please, do your exercises and spend some hours a day with minimal restriction around your chest. It has been suggested that the biggest cause of breast cancer is the restriction on the lymphatic drainage system from the long-term wearing of bras.

Massage

One of the more pleasurable lymphatic drainage processes is massage. However, many massage therapists and teaching institutions have such a lack of understanding of how the body is constructed that many of the massage strokes are carried out against the direction of the lymphatic flow.

The lymphatic system contains hundreds of extremely delicate nonreturn valves, and to massage the lymphatic fluid against the natural opening of these valves can seriously damage their one-way function. For correct lymphatic drainage, all firm massage strokes should go from the extremities toward the neck.

COLON CLEANSING

As suggested earlier, the lower digestive tract and colon can become very toxic due to incorrectly fermented foods, so cleaning the digestive tract is of paramount importance in any detoxification program. There is a tremendous amount of information available regarding colon-cleansing techniques and processes, some of which necessitate the flushing of the colon by inserting tubes into the rectum (colonics).

When we look at the construction of the body, and in particular, the way the sphincter muscle controls the anal opening, it is very easy to see that this muscle is a one-way valve. It is designed to allow movement from inside the body to the outside. To feed any object from the outside in through the anal opening is to totally distort and electrically damage the cells of the sphincter muscle. Under no circumstances do I recommend colonic flushing because of this potential electrical damage.

In addition, the inserting of the tube, in colonic flushing, has an extremely high chance of damaging another one-way valve system in the upper rectal cavity, the transverse rectal fold valve. These valve systems are electrically connected to the circuitry that governs the spasms of the levator anal muscle, which allows bowel movements, and other muscle groups within the rectum. Because they are also electrically connected to the upper colon cavities, electrical damage to a large portion of the colon is a high possibility.

The follicles on the inside of the colon cavity send an electrical message down to the valves of the anus and control the opening and closing. Any damage to the electrical function of this complex circuitry has the potential to promote the onset of colon cancer. Remember, cancer starts as an electrical malfunction.

Even though colonics are one of the methods used to reduce the risk of colon cancer, the possible electrical damage may outweigh the benefits. The entire colon system is constructed for the one-way movement. Anything other than this one-way movement is an extreme violation of nature's complex plumbing system, as well as a total distortion of the electrical interface between millions of cells.

There are many other ways to remove the buildup of semidecayed matter from the colon, but, sadly, many of them put the body under far too much physical stress, thereby causing electrical damage to massive amounts of cells within the colon. Any cleansing method that creates physical discomfort is electrical bombardment. Most drug-based diuretics fall into this category.

Many herbal concoctions can also have a powerful cleaning effect on the colon, and, unfortunately, a large percentage of herbal-based colon cleanse formulations do not take into consideration the electrical chaos that results from their action.

The object of a cleanse is to move all of the digested food matter through the colon as well as slowly softening and removing any built-up residue on the walls of the colon. At the same time, it is necessary to supply to the cells the nutrition needed to help rebuild any damage.

A successful, trauma-free colon cleanse, using products that enhance rather than damage the electrical function of the cells and that are formulated with the knowledge outlined in the following section, will take up to a year to complete. A colon cleanse cannot be done safely, quickly. The risk of causing extreme irritation and subsequently increasing the risk of colon cancer is very real.

Electrically Available Herbal Cleanse

Herbal formulations that are combined using the knowledge of the electrical matrix of the individual herbs and their combined action are of paramount importance in any colon cleansing and rebuilding procedure. After many years of studying the electrical matrix of herbs, the industry leaders now have electrically correct herbal formulations. Any herbal formulas created without an electrical understanding have the potential to cause more harm than good. Remember, as soon as you mix two of anything together, you change the electrical matrix and thus its behavior—and thereby its interface with everything else. If one herb has a diuretic effect and another a scouring action, putting the two together in the body may mean that neither function takes place. Thus the importance of knowing and understanding the electrical compatibility and the electrical function in anything we do to the body.

Traditional Chinese medicine holds that every disease that manifests in the human body originates from imbalances within the colon. With our modern food manufacturing methods and serious overindulgence in sugar and wheat, probably very few human beings in the Western world have healthy, nontoxic colons.

If you only took an electrically formulated herbal colon cleanse daily, like the one available from Avena Originals or Electrical Nutrition Professional (see Appendix A), you would be doing more to alleviate the toxic effects of modern living and eating than any other single thing you could possibly do. However, when combined with adequate levels of electrically correct hydration and at least thirty minutes a day of good physical lymphatic movement, you can exponentially decrease the future risk of disease manifestation and dramatically reduce any existing disease symptoms. The cleaning of the body's lymphatic drainage system and lower digestive tract is of paramount importance in returning the body to homeostasis (electrical harmony) and achieving a long, disease-free life.

There is not one disease that cannot be reversed. Your body desperately seeks its health and vitality. With a little bit of help on your behalf, it will respond beyond your wildest dreams.

ELECTRICALLY FORMULATED NUTRITIONAL SUPPORT

The dietary supplementation industry has enjoyed an exponential growth in the last ten years, despite the original negative rumblings from the pharmaceutical industry that supplements were not necessary. The same pharmaceutical industry now manufactures the raw material for the biggest percentage of supplements. The worldwide swing toward nutritional supplementation was apparently a market the pharmaceutical companies could not ignore. However, these pharmaceutical companies manufacture these nutritional supplements (which are predominantly those sold in drugstores and health-food stores) on the principles of traditional chemical medicine—by following the old paradigm of particle physics, not an electrical perspective. If our traditional scientific and pharmaceutical industries refuse to accept the leading-edge research into the electrical universe, the nutritional supplements being produced cannot be electrically available to the body.

As Albert Einstein said, "We cannot change the problems with the level of thinking that created them." Supplementation up until now has not worked very well. We are still sick and disease-ridden. We obviously need a new level of thinking and a new source of nutritional supplements that are "electrically available" to the body. Supplements should be formulated with the understanding of the whole electrical process.

A small number of scientists are researching the electrical compatibility of different herbs and minerals and their correct electrical interface with the cells in our bodies; their work is at the cutting edge of nutritional science. Using electrical compatibility knowledge, these researchers have formulated some of the world's most advanced "electrically available" natural nutritional supplements. We now have health-giving products that act the way nature and our bodies work—electrically. (See Appendix A for information on obtaining these products.) These products and their ability to interface with our bodies to detoxify and reverse the degeneration that we call disease are light-years ahead of anything we ever had previously. We are talking about a completely different set of rules—electrical rules—that before now we did not know existed.

Before this "electrically available" knowledge, the industry standard for the absorbability of nutritional supplements had been around 10 percent. That is why many doctors and others have said that taking supplements is a waste of time. It is only in the last few years that electrically formulated products, with an availability to the cells that at times exceeds 90 percent, have been available through mail-order health clubs and other high-end retail health professionals.

Ten years ago, we had no knowledge of the importance of electrical availability in anything, let alone our food or supplementation. Quantum physics is working toward the realization that everything interfaces with everything else on an energy level. Doctors and nutritionists who close their minds to what we know about electrical availability and the wholesale destruction of the body caused by the electrical damage from what we thought was food are ignoring current scientific knowledge.

It is sad but true that change is slow to take hold. This is especially true in the health and medical fields. History shows us that change is even slower when some new knowledge comes along that requires a complete 180-degree turn in our thinking, and we have to get our minds around a completely different set of parameters.

One such change that was slow to take hold occurred in the middle of the nineteenth century. John Robbins tells the following story:

> Ignaz Semmelweis, a young obstetrician who delivered babies in a famous Viennese hospital noticed women coming to give birth were sent to one of the hospital's two sections—the First Clinic, where obstetricians prevailed and medical students received training, or the Second Clinic, staffed entirely by midwives. Noticing that women were literally begging to be admitted to the Second Clinic, Semmelweis began to look carefully at the autopsy records from the two sections. What he discovered was that the death rate from puerperal fever [also called childbed fever] for women in the "doctor's" wards was more that four times higher than for women under the midwives' jurisdiction.
>
> Semmelweis, like other doctors of his time, had no idea that germs could cause disease. This was some twenty years before Joseph Lister would advance the use of antiseptics in surgery. But, in a moment of inspiration, he decreed that the medical students handling deliveries on his ward should wash their hands in a chlorine solution after dissecting corpses, and after each examination of a woman in the ward.

The results were outstanding. Before the hand washing, one out of every eight woman giving birth in the First Clinic had died of puerperal fever. But now the death rate dropped almost immediately to less than 1 in 100.

What do you think the reaction was when Semmelweis published the records of this spectacular success? Was he heralded and applauded, and his ideas immediately put into practice in all obstetrical clinics?

Not quite; orthodox obstetricians virtually declared war on the poor man, battering and insulting him at every opportunity. He was hounded from Vienna and eventually driven insane by the relentless attacks. He died without ever knowing that his views would eventually triumph, and thanks to his discoveries [or was it the midwives that he learned it from], puerperal fever would nearly disappear.

Why were such spectacular results dismissed by the medical establishment of the day? [Was it that] members of the medical establishment were at that time implacably resistant to any insinuation that their own practices were harming [women]?[1, 2]

We do now have available to us electrically formulated, electrically available supplements that are compatible with the body's electrical system (see Appendix A for information on where to obtain them). Consciousness is slowly changing, and it is up to us to take advantage of these advances.

FORTIFYING AGAINST ELECTROMAGNETIC FREQUENCIES (EMFs)

In Chapter 4 we discussed different forms of electromagnetic pollution and the effects of electromagnetic frequencies on our vitality and general health. As we become more industrialized and more technologically advanced, particularly in the personal electronics field, our environment is becoming ever more saturated with subtle forms of frequencies that have a potentially damaging effect on our body's electromagnetic system.

As a result of this very real and measurable bombardment, I have been very concerned about how we can fortify our body's electrical system so that disease states do not develop as a result of electromagnetic pollution. There are many theories of how best to achieve this fortification, and I suggest that those interested do their own research. However, on the basis of my research, I believe there are very few products or processes that are actually technologically advanced and have a measurable effect in their ability to reduce the effects of electromagnetic pollution on the body. I personally use a product called Q-Link, manufactured by Clarus International, as I believe this is one of the few products that has the technological sophistication and research backing to be an effective instrument. (See Appendix A for more information.)

Summary

To clean up your body and get it functioning at a higher level, you have to make some life-affirmative changes and integrate some of the suggestions in this chapter. For starters, you can increase your protein intake and daily consumption of fresh fruits and vegetables, cut out the grain (bread, cereals, pasta), and keep the proteins and carbohydrates separate. Then start the process of cleaning up the body with an electrically available colon cleanse and electrically available water. Increase the amount of movement per day and include up-and-down movement on an electrically tuned mini-trampoline or some vigorous free dance. To top it off, supplement your diet with some high-tech electrically formulated enzymes, herbs, and minerals to make up for the lack in modern food sources.

None of these suggestions in isolation will do everything for you, but put together in balance they all add to the potential of each other, so the sum becomes very much greater than the individual components. This is the basis of electrical nutrition and vibrational medicine.

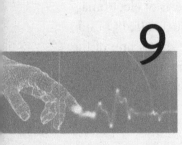

9

Life — An Electrical Reality

In order for us to really feel at peace and in harmony, we first have to find that harmony within. Once we find that harmony, it then has as a ripple effect, rippling out into our relationships, our families, our communities, our jobs. As everything in this universe is energy, and all energy communicates with all other energy, it makes sense that if we focus on harmonizing our own reality first, then our energy will start radiating health and vitality and attract to it similar energy.

In my last book, *Journey to Truth*, I discussed many energy concepts and suggested that energy mastery can give us the keys to life, love, wealth, and health. Everything is interrelated and connected.

We continue here to share specific, practical, self-help information. If you choose to implement this knowledge in your life, you will indeed benefit dramatically. Life can become more harmonious, love can bloom, wealth can start to flow, and health—the starting point of it all—can continue to blossom in ever-increasing states of vitality and life-exuding bliss.

It is said that there are a million causes of disease, but in fact there is only one cause of disease, and that is electrical malfunction. On the other hand, the electrical malfunction can have a million different causes. This is obvious when we accept and understand the concept of an electrical universe. From an electrical perspective, everything we do, feel, and touch, and everything that everybody else does has an impact on the frequencies of energy that are then released into this electrical universe of ours.

THE UNIVERSAL SOUP BOWL OF ENERGY

Our electrical universe is like a great soup bowl, and every thought, word, and deed; every ounce of pollution; every bit of everything adds to the components of our soup bowl. We are not immune to the effects of all these different frequencies because our physicality, our emotions, our actions, and our thoughts are all part of the ingredients of the soup. Yet within this gigantic mixture, our consciousness—or the group of frequencies that condense into who we are—has an ability to govern which subtle frequencies impact us. However, like a radio, we can only be receptive to (or conscious of) a frequency that is being transmitted if we ourselves are tuned in to that particular frequency. For example, a radio that is tuned to the AM band cannot pick up and play the song that is being transmitted by the FM station.

Our cellular structure—its behavior, function, and health—is totally governed by the frequency contained within it. Everything in this universe works with exactly the same laws, which are sometimes referred to as natural law, or cosmic law. A more accurate understanding would be to say that this universe works on the laws of *energy*.

When we look at how energy manifests, we find that the lower the frequency, the more dense or solid is the physicality. The frequency change to a lower vibratory rate manifests as increasing density in the cellular structure, and that is the start of all disease. As we load onto ourselves any disharmonic frequency, whether it be in the form of emotional or physical stress, chemical toxins, emotional reactivities, lifestyle choices, and so on, we promote the densification of our cellular structure.

This electrical loading severely restricts the electrical circuitry or the energy flow through our body's subtle electrical circuits. As the frequency drops, the flow is reduced, the cells become compacted, the tissues become more dense, we tighten up, there is less blood flow and lymphatic drainage, the bowels constrict, the chest tightens, the heart constricts, and so forth.

As all these physical restrictions happen, names of disease are given to the physical body's reactions to these constrictions of energy flow. The symptoms we rush off to our doctors or physiotherapists for are all caused by this physical energetic reactivity. All malfunctions and illness in the body can be traced energetically to an electrical malfunction, and can be perceived by those consciously aware of the subtle frequencies.

There are many therapists who, with little understanding of this energy communication, label it as psychic ability or medical intuitiveness or use other so-called New Age terminology. In fact, what is taking place is a very natural energy communication, something that is constantly happening among all aspects of this cosmos at all times.

It is not too difficult to learn to enhance your conscious awareness of this energy communication. Just as a radio can receive a transmission from a radio station if it is tuned into the same (right) frequency, so too can we tune into the frequency of what we are. Likewise, most of the New Age so-called special abilities and what some would term spiritual gifts are also the same perfectly natural, everyday energy communications. This conscious communication can be mastered by anybody willing to invest in the time to learn. It is not a special gift.

We are energy, and our energy is interfacing with all other energy at all times. We just have to become conscious of it. There is not one part of the body that is not affected by everything we do and everything everybody else does. There are times when we allow our behavior to be directly influenced by the frequency of energy that has been transmitted by somebody else.

For example, when people get into their emotions and pour out their anger, that anger is transmitted as a frequency of energy. Three thousand miles away, if somebody who is also experiencing his emotions happens to be on the same frequency, zap! That person takes on the energy that was transmitted. Now that person is really angry, and his energy is sucking in any frequency that matches. Remember, birds of a feather flock together, or in modern language, energy is received on the same frequency that it was transmitted on. The person 3,000 miles away is now out of control and picking up more and more disharmonic frequencies from many different people until he explodes, picks up a gun, and blows somebody away. Shock! Horror! What a bad person. Let's judge him, lock him up, and throw the key away.

Perhaps the lesson for us here is that the person who exploded and blew somebody else away with a gun just *rephysicalized* all the disharmonic frequencies that were transmitted by the rest of us. Yes, he may have pulled the trigger, but who produced the frequencies of energy that were the disharmony he responded to? The universe is a closed electrical circuit. All frequency moves from physical to energy and then has to be rephysicalized—the circuit has to be completed.

This concept of rephysicalizing energy parallels the Christian saying "What you sow, so shall you reap" and the Eastern concept of the laws of karma. It is time to look beyond our limited perceptions, understand another reality, embrace another consciousness—that of the electrical universe—and then we may be able to see and understand that we are all one.

THERE IS NO MAGIC PILL

Everybody is looking for that magic pill, therapist, or one technique that will cure all aches, pains, and illnesses (physical and emotional). Very few people are truly committed to putting a real investment of energy or time into their health and well-being. Almost everybody is looking for an answer outside of themselves.

There is no reason why we should be unhealthy, in pain, or suffering in any way. Almost every dis-ease is reversible if you are willing to make that investment in yourself and a commitment to really becoming healthy. But you have to start with yourself!

It was said that the Kingdom of Heaven (which could be considered to be the body) is guarded by the pearly gates. The only pearls in our bodies are our teeth. Is this a metaphor that is telling us that our electrical frequency, our health, and our enlightenment is indexed to what comes in and what goes out of these pearly gates—the mouth? Everything we take in through our mouth and everything we express (thought, word, and deed) is a frequency of energy, and energy shapes everything—energy *is* everything. Our connection with all that is always has been right here in front of us when we look in the mirror. It is not out there somewhere—we are it.

LIFE'S EXPERIENCES

It is fascinating to look at life's experiences (both good and bad) as gifts. And it is healthy to look at illness/accidents/disease as gifts in disguise. They are often a wake-up call, a powerful message for us to open our eyes and see what we are doing to ourselves, to look at our habits, patterns, and conditionings and reassess them. Are these beliefs really in my best interest? Am I really all that I can be, or am I holding back in some way?

Certain physical states manifest in our bodies because we have been deaf to subtle messages that have been recurring over and over again. So the body finally realizes that you need a bigger hammer to make you see the woes of your ways. Louise Hay, author of *You Can Heal Your Life* (Hay House), and Caroline Myss, author of *Anatomy of the Spirit* (Harmony Books) have explained in their books how to look beyond the physical to other emotional, mental, spiritual and energy reasons for the development of illness.

It is important that we are not too simplistic in our analysis and that we understand that each individual has his or her own unique set of life circumstances and conditions. We should never put anyone in a box or assume that because they have developed, for example, stomach problems that it is because they have un-dealt-with emotional issues, or because someone has AIDS they have fallen into the victim mode or been sexually promiscuous, or if I broke my foot it is because I am not walking my truth, and so on.

Sometimes "stuff happens"! Everyone has transmitted disharmonic frequencies, and sometimes we are just rephysicalizing that disharmony if we happened to be tuned to a particular frequency at a particular time. Analysis often becomes our paralysis. It is much more advantageous to accept what has happened, learn from it, and move on with our lives, focusing on what can help us to live a full and healthy life. Follow your bliss!

Remember, we get a very good look at where we come from when we drive our car down the road backward, but all hell will break out in front of us because we are not watching where we are going. Life is a forward path—a path that gives us experiences. We learn to accept these experiences by not taking them too seriously. It is only then that we can open up to the full joy, bliss, and harmony that is available.

It is imperative that we challenge our own belief parameters about health and well-being. It is necessary to learn from our mistakes—to not dwell on them and use them as excuses to get stuck in the bog, but rather to accept them and move on. This cannot be emphasized enough. The keys to good health are to look, to see, to understand, to accept, and *to move on*. Granted, this is not always easy to do, but it is possible. This is one of the things we address in our workshops held around the world.

In my many years of clinical experience, it has become obvious that it is possible to alleviate most conditions with advanced vibrational medicine techniques, but inevitably people seem to go back to their old ways and the original problem recurs. It is only possible to give people so much information and so much assistance (physically, emotionally, and spiritually); ultimately it is up to them to use their willpower to actually take the bull by the horns and really make a difference.

That is why I do not like the term "healer." Nobody can heal anybody else. Practitioners can assist in many ways. We can present people with a mirror so they can see themselves. We can alleviate the stress loading on the cells. We can recharge the batteries, so to speak, and correct many electrical malfunctions. We can physically mend bones, sew up cuts, or remove malfunctioning parts when there is no other option. We can explain nutrition and the importance of movement and how the body works. But what it really comes down to in the end is one's determination to heal oneself. We cannot *heal* anyone—we can only assist someone on his or her own healing journey.

CLEARING THE CELLULAR HARD DRIVE

All of our life experiences are stored in our cellular memory as frequencies of energy. What we consciously remember could be described as only that which appears on the screen (of the computer); everything else is stored on the hard drive, as it were. It is all there. We may not be able to see it all at one time, but it is there.

It is possible to reduce the stress loading on our cellular structure by deleting some of the files that are no longer of any use, and we can also "defrag" (or clean up) the hard drive or simply stop adding so many files to our already full memory.

There are many different ways to clean up our hard drives (our cellular bodies). The long way is to pull up every old file, read through it, and then throw it in the recycle bin. This is very laborious and time consuming as well as very tiring energetically. And often we go through this whole process, the old file ends up in the recycle bin, and we forget that it actually still exists on our hard drive, since we have not completely removed it from our cellular memory, only filed it in another part of the system.

Many emotional release techniques and psychoanalytical practices in the Western world resemble this way of dealing with old files. Often a lot of time and energy is spent on bringing back up all the old files and going through them with a fine-tooth comb—actually reexperiencing the scenarios and reprogramming them onto the cellular structure once more without actually changing them in any way or deleting them, which was supposedly the aim of the process in the first place!

There are other ways to safely remove unuseful files from your cellular memory. The aim of vibrational medicine is to encourage people to learn how to raise their vibrational frequency so that they can transmute any disharmonic frequency contained within their cellular structure into a harmonic one. Vibrational medicine and many of these concepts are taught worldwide by the International Institute of Vibrational Wellness. (See Appendix A for more information.)

Transmuting Disharmonic Frequencies

Imagine your life force as a small, smoldering campfire. If somebody comes along and dumps a wheelbarrowful of wet leaves on your small campfire, the leaves would probably smother the fire and snuff it out! And it really does feel like that sometimes. We struggle to keep our own fire burning, and it certainly knocks us around when somebody comes along and dumps on us with a lot of anger or any emotional outpouring of energy, or even when things just do not seem to be going right. If we are only a small smoldering campfire, these experiences will affect us dramatically.

The aim is not to get rid of the wet leaves in our lives—they exist. The objective is to build up our own fire into a roaring bonfire so that those wet leaves no longer have a negative effect on us but rather can be used as fuel for our fire. The wet leaves dry up in our heat and then act as fuel! We can transmute what would initially be considered disharmonic energy into beneficial energy.

Similarly, with our life experiences, we can choose to see them as negative and let them create disharmony in our lives, or we can transmute them into a positive experience—learn from them and take those life experiences and use them to benefit ourselves. For example, the gift of a heart attack may well be a total turnaround of diet and lifestyle, which may enable you to enjoy and benefit greatly from this experience called life!

In order to transmute these so-called negative experiences into positive ones, we have to build our own fires first. We have to work on our own self-esteem, and fortify our own systems by supplementing our diets with electrically available nutrients, eating the right foods in the right combinations, being aware of the factors in our lives that create stress loading on our cellular structure, and ensuring that our body, heart, and soul receive as much nourishment as possible, which would include joyful movement, lots of loving, and reflective quiet times.

One could use the analogy of a truck laden with rocks struggling up a steep hill. We are that truck, life is that steep incline, and the rocks are our accumulation of stress and experiences that weigh us down. The truck can only take so much, and there are only a limited number of repairs that can be done until it can no longer do the job it was designed to do.

We are the same. Our bodies can only take so much. There are only so many pills we can take to suppress the pain, which is a symptom of an electrical malfunction. If we do not address the causes of the malfunction and take some of the loading off, we, too, soon stop working completely. To return to full health we have to reduce the load. Sometimes this requires us to make some very difficult lifestyle choices, but that is the experience and the joy of living—learning to make these choices.

ELECTRICAL HEALTH—YOUR NEW OCCUPATION

Staying healthy and happy is a full-time job. It does not have to be a laborious, difficult, or painful process. It can be fun and can be integrated into your present lifestyle. It is a conscious choice we can all make to be more aware about what we put into our bodies, how our bodies react, how we feel in certain situations, and what our needs truly are. What is it that gives us joy, that makes us feel happy and healthy?

Health and happiness are not found in a pill or in a doctor's consultation room. True health and happiness is a learned process, and the key is inside you. The way to find it is to have determination and the will to invest your time and energy in yourself. And remember, follow your bliss. Make each moment a joyful one, each mouthful of food a nourishing one, each experience a chance to learn something new, and each connection with another an opportunity to share love, to be love, and to experience this experience called life without limits, to love without limits, to be without limits.

But remember, we cannot share what we do not have, so start with loving and accepting yourself. Look after your body. It is your only vehicle of experience this time around. Electrical nutrition is the key to electrical harmony. Electrical harmony is the key to your bliss, health, wealth, and enlightenment. And do not forget—seriousness is outlawed.

Enjoy!

In Light and Love,
DENIE AND SHELLEY

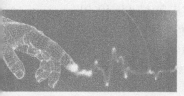

APPENDIX A.

Resources

We have discussed many topics and analyzed many ideas. People continually ask me where to obtain the electrically formulated, electrically available nutritional supplements we have mentioned. As a result of being in the natural health industry for more than twenty years, I have come into contact with some amazing products and equipment, have been party to the development of various supplements and health tools, and have tried many products from the world's best formulators and producers.

Most of the good high tech-products are available only through network marketing organizations and small, specialized health clubs. This can result in therapists and clinics having difficulty supplying these products to their clients.

I remember years ago there was an advertisement on television for Remington shavers. The owner of Remington shavers appeared in this ad and stated with a big smile on his face, while holding a Remington shaver, "I found the product so good—I bought the company." It was an award-winning ad that catapulted Remington's sales dramatically.

Well, I guess I could be compared in some ways to the owner of the Remington shaver company, since as a result of the increasing requests I received from doctors, therapists, and health clinics to supply them these high-tech products, I literally "bought the company." In other words, I have obtained the licenses and marketing agreements to a range of what I perceive to be the best products in the world—all created with the understanding of the electrical interface between the molecules and formulated so that they are electrically available to the body. Along with a group of investors I pulled together, I started my company, Electrical Nutrition Professional, with the express purposes of making the best of the best available to all health professionals. It is a wholesale-only company that sells to licensed health-care professionals and is not involved with retail sales.

Information on this and other companies is provided below. (This is by no means a complete list of companies that provide electrically available products, but it is certainly a start.)

www.vibrationalmedicine.com
Tel: 310-821-4703
For information about the International Institute of Vibrational Wellness, which teaches vibrational medicine, personal growth, and health and awareness seminars worldwide; Denie Hiestand's autobiography *Journey to Truth*; and Denie Hiestand's Wellness Clinic.

www.electrical-nutrition.net
Tel: 1-800-856-6448 or 310-577-2575
For electrically available, electrically formulated natural health products for health professionals.

www.avenaoriginals.com
Tel: 1-800-207-2239
For electrically available, electrically formulated natural health supplements for individuals.

www.rbcnow.com/vibrationalmedicine.asp
Tel: 1-877-254-8300 or 425-827-7773
For microhydrin to help make water electrically available.

www.clarus.com
For scientific studies on Q-Links (to fortify the electromagnetic field of the body).

www.karikaas.co.nz
For yogurt containing the B.O.D. strain of bifidus and high-quality cheeses.

Email drglum@attglobal.net
For html versions of the books *Calling of an Angel* and *Full Disclosure.*

www.dorway.com
For information on aspartame.
Mission Possible International
Contact: Mrs. Betty Martini
Email: bettym19@mindspring.com
Tel: 770-242-2599

www.sunsentpress.com
For Dr. Robert's book *Defense Against Alzheimer's Disease.*

www.newtrendspublishing.com
For Sally Fallon and Mary G. Enig's book *Nourishing Traditions.*

TaeBo videos can be obtained by calling 1-877-BBTAEBO (228-2326).

An electrically available source of tocotrienols is available to health professionals under the name of Protein Power, from Electrical Nutrition Professional, www.electrical-nutrition.net (1-800-856-6448 or 310-577-2575), or to individuals under the name of TOCO, through Avena Originals, www.avenaoriginals.com (1-800-207-2239 or 403-314-2351).

Latero Flora is available to health professionals through Electrical Nutrition Professional, www.electrical-nutrition.net (1-800-856-6448 or 310-577-2575) or to individuals through Avena Originals, www.avenaoriginals.com (1-800-207-2239 or 403-314-2351).

New Zealand Colostrum is available to health professionals through Electrical Nutrition Professional, www.electrical-nutrition.net (1-800-856-6448 or 310-577-2575), or to individuals through Avena Originals, www.avenaoriginals.com (1-800-207-2239 or 403-314-2351).

Electrically available herbs and supplements can be obtained by contacting Electrical Nutrition Professional, www.electrical-nutrition.net (1-800-856-6448 or 310-577-2575) who wholesale these electrically formulated combinations to health professionals, or Avena Originals, www.avenaoriginals.com (1-800-207-2239 or 403-314-2351), who sell these formulations to individuals.

Come Alive, Dr. Bernard Jensen, DC, Ph.D. Available from www.avenaoriginals.com, or by calling 1-800-207-2239 or 403-314-2351.

The B.O.D. strain of bifidus is sold under the name of Latero Flora and is available to health professionals through Electrical Nutrition Professional, www.electrical-nutrition.net (1-800-856-6448 or 310-577-2575), or through Avena Originals if you are an individual, www.avenaoriginals.com (1-800-207-2239 or 403-314-2351). Visit also www.karikaas.com for information about a new yogurt that contains the B.O.D. strain of bifidus.

Friendly Flora, *L. salivarius* and *L. plantarium* are available to health professionals under the name of Digestive Flora, from Electrical Nutrition Professional, www.electrical-nutrition.net (1-800-856-6448 or 310-577-2575), or to individuals under the name of Friendly Flora through Avena Originals, www.avenaoriginals.com (1-800-207-2239 or 403-314-2351).

Microhydrin is available through Royal Body Care, a network marketing company. Call Alia, an independent distributor of Microhydrin at 1-877-254-8300 or 425-827-7773, or visit www.rbcnow.com/vibrationalmedicine.asp. Or you can also use a product called Cell Food to oxygenate your water. Cell Food is available to health professionals through Electrical Nutrition Professional, www.electrical-nutrition.net (1-800-856-6448 or 310-577-2575), or to individuals through Avena Originals, www.avenaoriginals.com (1-800-207-2239 or 403-314-2351).

The electrically tuned rebounder is available to health professionals through Electrical Nutrition Professional, www.electrical-nutrition.net (1-800-856-6448 or 310-577-2575), or through Avena Originals if you are an individual, www.avenaoriginals.com (1-800-207-2239 or 403-314-2351).

The electrically available herbal cleanse is available to health professionals under the name of Herbal Cleanse from Electrical Nutrition Professional, www.electrical-nutrition.net (1-800-856-6448 or 310-577-2575), or to individuals under the name of Herb Cocktail, through Avena Originals, www.avenaoriginals.com (1-800-207-2239 or 403-314-2351).

Q-Links, manufactured by Clarus International: For more scientific research, visit www.clarus.com. Q-Links are also available to health professionals from Electrical Nutrition Professional, www.electrical-nutrition.net (1-800-856-6448 or 310-577-2575), or to individuals from Avena Originals, www.avenaorginals.com (1-800-207-2239 or 403-314-2351).

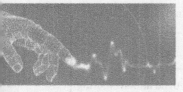

APPENDIX B.

Sample Electrical Menus and Seven Steps to Good Health

Many people think that if they implement the electrical nutrition concepts, their diet will be very limited. This is definitely not the case. Here, we give you some examples of what we eat daily to help you get started. Of course, you are invited to be creative and try some combinations and ideas of your own.

The most important rule of thumb is: Eat food the way nature made it. Keep it simple, keep it fresh, keep it raw. Eating raw food may be a stretch, but try to integrate this slowly into your diet. Cooking is a preserving process and slows fermentation. Raw food is more easily fermented and gives greater life force. Choosing organic sources is highly recommended. Use your powerful sense of smell to let you know whether your food is fresh.

W E E K   O N E
Monday

Breakfast	Take an electrically available herbal cleanse[1] when you first wake up, one-half hour before eating. Then eat a banana or other fruit or berries. Mix fruit with whole-milk natural yogurt if desired. Add a dash of maple syrup or raw unheated honey[2] (optional). You can also add a raw, fertile free-range egg and some raw/fresh cream (optional).
Snack	Protein supplement[3] to supply necessary components missing from today's foodstuffs. *Or* a piece of fruit.
Lunch	European-style (choose natural cheeses with no added coloring) cheese or cheese made with raw milk and grapes .
Snack	An organic apple or orange, or a few soft or soaked nuts. *Or* a power drink—such as organic bovine colostrum,[4] shaken with half a cup of water, and a raw organic egg (optional) and a dash of maple syrup or unheated honey (optional). Add extra enzymes[5] to enhance digestion.
Dinner	Filet mignon or other top quality cut (6–8 oz.) (or raw if possible), portobello mushrooms, and onions cooked lightly in butter; green beans lightly steamed.
Dessert (optional)	Whole dates, cut in half, pitted, and filled with cream cheese. (You won't need too many, as these are very rich.)

[1] Herbal Cleanse from Electrical Nutrition Professional (ENP), or Herb Cocktail from Avena Originals.

[2] Heating destroys many of the natural enzymes in honey. Use raw unheated honey if possible.

[3] Protein Power from ENP, or TOCO from Avena Originals.

[4] Symbiotics Colostrum, available from ENP or Avena Originals.

[5] High-grade enzymes, available from ENP or Avena Originals.

W E E K O N E
Tuesday

Breakfast	Herbal cleanse Fruit and/or yogurt
Snack	Protein supplement and/or piece of fruit
Lunch	Tuna salad *Or* cheese and grapes
Snack	Fruits or nuts *Or* a power drink
Dinner	Fresh salmon raw or seared very lightly in butter, asparagus tips very lightly steamed, and a raw tomato
Dessert	Hot drink made with milk (using raw milk if possible) — hot chocolate or decaf coffee — and a piece of organic sugar-free chocolate (get one sweetened with cane juice but NO aspartame!) or some powdered raw carob beans

WEEK ONE	
Wednesday	
Breakfast	Herbal cleanse Fruit and/or yogurt
Snack	Protein supplement and/or piece of fruit
Lunch	Boiled eggs and carrots *Or* wrap some ham around eggs cut into quarters *Or* a Cobb salad *Or* cheese and grapes
Snack	Fruit or nuts *Or* a power drink
Dinner	Roast potatoes with butter (raw organic butter if possible), vegetables or a salad (organic)
Dessert	Some fresh organic grapes

W E E K O N E	
Thursday	
Breakfast	Herbal cleanse Fruit and/or yogurt
Snack	Protein supplement and/or piece of fruit
Lunch	Potato salad (Use the extra potatoes from last night's dinner to make a potato salad for lunch. Add a balsamic vinegar/olive oil dressing and some finely chopped pickles or red onion.) *Or* cheese and grapes
Snack	Fruit or nuts *Or* a power drink
Dinner	Lamb chops with minted peas and carrots (make sure the lamb is real lamb and not mutton—best to get New Zealand or Australian lamb). Cook lightly. *Or* raw ground lamb mixed with raw eggs, cream, butter, and unheated honey.
Dessert	Glass of red wine and a piece of soft cheese, such as Brie or Camembert. (One glass of red wine, organic if possible, will aid digestion; however, more than one will stop fermentation.)

WEEK ONE	
Friday	
Breakfast	Herbal cleanse Fruit and/or yogurt
Snack	Protein supplement and/or piece of fruit
Lunch	Swiss cheese and pickle. (Eat a variety of different natural cheeses that have no added coloring. Make sure the pickle is natural with no MSG or added sulfites.) *Or* cheese and grapes
Snack	Fruit or nuts *Or* a power drink
Dinner	Quiche *Or* if you really want to go totally raw, make up a mixture of raw eggs and cream mixed with unheated raw honey, butter, and some raw ground meat.
Dessert	Coconut apricot balls (grind dried apricots through hand grinder, rather than a food processor, and roll in coconut)

W E K   O N E
Saturday

Breakfast	Herbal cleanse Fruit and/or yogurt
Snack	Protein supplement and/or piece of fruit
Lunch	Avocado salad. Or cut the avocado in half, drip some balsamic vinegar and olive oil in the center, plus salt and pepper. *Or* cheese and grapes
Snack	Fruit or nuts *Or* a power drink
Dinner	Cut free-range chicken breasts into pieces and lightly fry in butter (or eat raw if possible). Eat with lightly steamed/raw vegetables and/or a salad.
Dessert	Strawberries dipped in carob

W E E K   O N E
Sunday

Brunch	Bacon and eggs. Remember not to have the toast or hash browns. *Or* cheese and grapes
Snack	Latté, with whole milk (One coffee per day is OK, as long as you have it with whole milk or cream. This helps to reduce the stripping effect of the coffee.)
Dinner	Barbecue (summertime) or a meat casserole (winter), or a feast of raw meat to stick with the raw-food diet.
Dessert	Raw ice cream made with organic milk, cream, berries of choice, juice of a lemon, juice of a lime, and some unheated honey to sweeten. Beat together, by hand if possible and then freeze until cold and semi-solid.

W E E K   T W O

Monday

Breakfast	Herbal cleanse Fruit and/or yogurt
Snack	Protein supplement and/or piece of fruit
Lunch	Soup and salad. Make sure the soup does not contain noodles or pasta. And remember, no bread or crackers. Or simply a salad by itself. *Or* cheese and grapes
Snack	Fruit or nuts *Or* a power drink
Dinner	Tuna raw or lightly seared, with asparagus tips (lightly steamed) and a raw tomato. Cut the tuna into thin slices and dip into a mixture of wheat-free soya sauce and wasabi.
Dessert	Raisin and pecan balls (grind raisins through hand grinder, rather than a food processor, and roll in ground pecans or walnuts)

WEEK TWO	
Tuesday	
Breakfast	Herbal cleanse Fruit and/or yogurt
Snack	Protein supplement and/or piece of fruit
Lunch	Camembert cheese & nashi pear. Cut into thin slices, eat together. *Or* cheese and grapes
Snack	Fruit or nuts *Or* a power drink
Dinner	Buffalo or venison burgers without the bun. Lightly cook the burgers (or eat raw if you can), add tomato, pickle, lettuce, etc.
Dessert	Peaches and whipped cream

W E E K   T W O
W e d n e s d a y

Breakfast	Herbal cleanse Fruit and/or yogurt
Snack	Protein supplement and/or piece of fruit
Lunch	Tomato & mozzarella salad. Thinly slice tomatoes and mozzarella, sprinkle chopped basil on top with balsamic vinegar and olive oil, salt and pepper *Or* cheese and grapes
Snack	Fruit or nuts *Or* a power drink
Dinner	Your favorite bean dish (make sure beans are thoroughly soaked and cooked). Or a raw fresh green salad.
Dessert	Glass of red wine and a slice of soft cheese. (One glass of red wine, organic if possible, will aid digestion; however, more than one will stop fermentation.)

W E E K   T W O
Thursday

Breakfast	Herbal cleanse Fruit and/or yogurt
Snack	Protein supplement and/or piece of fruit
Lunch	Cheddar cheese, pickles, and dried red meat (salami/bundesfleish) *Or* cheese and grapes
Snack	Fruit or nuts *Or* a power drink
Dinner	Rack of lamb (preferably New Zealand or Australian lamb), cooked for about 35 minutes in the oven at about 350 degrees (cook less if you like it more raw), serve with peas and carrots and mint sauce. Or a raw meal of ground lamb, eggs, butter, cream, and unheated honey.
Dessert	Natural fruit dessert (hand-pressed fruits, sweetened with honey and lemon juice, and frozen)

W E K   T W O

Friday

Breakfast	Herbal cleanse Fruit and/or yogurt
Snack	Protein supplement and/or piece of fruit
Lunch	Avocado salad, or avocado cut in half with balsamic vinegar/olive oil dressing *Or* cheese and grapes
Snack	Fruit or nuts *Or* a power drink
Dinner	Raw white fish, marinated in lime juice and salt (for at least 4 hours). Mix with whole coconut milk, finely chopped onions, tomato, and garlic, and serve on lettuce leaves.
Dessert	Hot chocolate, chai tea, or decaf coffee. Add some unheated honey for extra sweetness.

WEEK TWO	
Saturday	
Breakfast	Herbal cleanse Fruit and/or yogurt
Snack	Protein supplement and/or piece of fruit
Lunch	Omelette—your choice of ingredients. (Remember, no bread or potatoes.) *Or* cheese and grapes
Snack	Fruit or nuts *Or* a power drink
Dinner	Filet mignon (or other good quality steak), with mushrooms, onions, and cream cheese, served with asparagus and a raw tomato. Thinly slice the meat and lightly stir-fry with the onions and mushrooms (or eat raw if desired). Add the cream cheese just at the end, before serving.
Dessert	Raspberry parfait (fresh fruit folded into stiffly beaten egg whites, sweetened with honey and lemon juice)

W E E K   T W O
Sunday

Brunch	Bacon and eggs (choose good quality bacon and organic eggs if possible). Add a raw tomato too. Or a raw egg mixture. *Or* cheese and grapes
Snack	Latté with whole milk (One coffee per day is OK, as long as you have it with whole milk or cream. This helps to reduce the stripping effect of the coffee.)
Dinner	Potatoes fried in butter, like French fries. Boil potatoes and then finish them off by frying in butter. Cook extra for lunch tomorrow.
Dessert	Fresh pineapple

W E E K T H R E E	
Monday	
Breakfast	Herbal cleanse Fruit and/or yogurt
Snack	Protein supplement and/or piece of fruit
Lunch	Potato salad. Use extra potatoes from last night's dinner to make a potato salad. *Or* cheese and grapes
Snack	Fruit or nuts *Or* a power drink
Dinner	Chicken—boil free-range chicken thighs in water with fresh ginger and basil (until soft and tender. Do not overcook. Or eat raw if desired). Drain, serve with fresh mixed organic vegetables and an organic olive oil and rice vinegar dressing. Add Celtic sea salt and freshly ground pepper.
Dessert	Fresh mango slices

W E E K   T H R E E
Tuesday

Breakfast	Herbal cleanse Fruit and/or yogurt
Snack	Protein supplement and/or piece of fruit
Lunch	Cheese and grapes (Stick with your favorite European cheese or good quality American—no added color.)
Snack	Fruit or nuts *Or* a power drink
Dinner	Salmon (raw or lightly seared in butter) with some cream cheese on top, sprinkled with green onions, served with lightly steamed or raw green beans. Add butter to the beans afterward.
Dessert	Almond date balls. Grind almonds through hand grinder, take the pits out of the dates and fill with ground almonds.

W E E K T H R E E	
Wednesday	
Breakfast	Herbal cleanse Fruit and/or yogurt
Snack	Protein supplement and/or piece of fruit
Lunch	Egg salad. Boil eggs, let cool, add tomato, cucumber, and other salad ingredients, with balsamic/olive oil dressing. *Or* raw egg mixture *Or* cheese and grapes
Snack	Fruit or nuts *Or* a power drink
Dinner	Buffalo or venison steak—lightly fried in butter or raw if possible, with a raw fresh green salad
Dessert	Glass of red wine and a slice of soft white cheese (One glass of red wine, organic if possible, will aid digestion; however, more than one will stop fermentation.)

W E E K   T H R E E

Thursday	
Breakfast	Herbal cleanse Fruit and/or yogurt
Snack	Protein supplement and/or piece of fruit
Lunch	Chicken salad (for example a Caesar salad with chicken, but not croutons) *Or* cheese and grapes
Snack	Fruit or nuts *Or* a power drink
Dinner	Sweet potatoes baked in the oven, cut thinly with layers of onions and butter. Cook at 350 degrees until potatoes are soft. Serve with salad or steamed vegetables.
Dessert	Dried unsulfured apricots dipped in carob

W E E K   T H R E E
Friday

Breakfast	Herbal cleanse Fruit and/or yogurt
Snack	Protein supplement and/or piece of fruit
Lunch	Potato salad—use extra potatoes from the night before or order one at the restaurant. A light mayonnaise is fine, otherwise try using olive oil and balsamic vinegar. *Or* cheese and grapes
Snack	Fruit or nuts *Or* a power drink
Dinner	Lightly cooked or raw chicken and lightly steamed/raw vegetables
Dessert	Hot chocolate, chai tea, or decaf coffee (with raw milk or organic milk)

W E E K T H R E E	
Saturday	
Breakfast	Herbal cleanse Fruit and/or yogurt
Snack	Protein supplement and/or piece of fruit
Lunch	Omelette—your choice of ingredients (Remember, no bread or potatoes)—or raw egg mixture *Or* cheese and grapes
Snack	Fruit or nuts *Or* a power drink
Dinner	Filet or steak—simple, plain, raw if possible or lightly seared, with lightly steamed vegetables
Dessert	Berries and fresh whipped cream

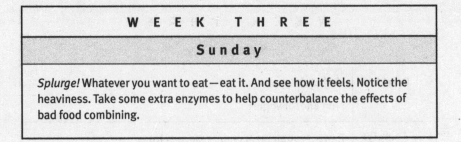

For those who wish to be more adventurous in the kitchen we highly recommend that you try some of the recipes in *Nourishing Traditions* (by Sally Fallon and Mary G. Enig, Ph.D., New Trends Publishing, 1999; www.newtrendspublishing.com or 1-877-707-1776). Remember not to mix your crude proteins (meat) and your crude carbohydrates (potatoes).

SEVEN STEPS TO GOOD HEALTH

Not everyone has the personality or willpower to suddenly change old patterns and shift 180 degrees into a new way of eating and living. We suggest that you take one step at a time. When you feel ready, try one or as many of the suggestions outlined below and see how you feel. The proof of the pudding is in the eating, so give it a go (as we say in New Zealand), and find out what makes you feel healthier and full of vitality.

1. *Separate your crude proteins and crude carbohydrates.* When you eat a meal, eat the protein (meat, fish, eggs, cheese, milk, cream, beans, nuts) with vegetables or a salad. If you want a carbohydrate meal, eat potatoes with vegetables or a salad. Make sure you have plenty of electrically available protein sources.

2. *Cut out all grains.* Do not eat any bread, pasta, doughnuts, pizza, cereals, cookies, or rice.

3. *Drink electrically alive water.* Collect your water from an underground water supply, a fresh-flowing river, a waterfall, or add Microhydrin or Cell Food to your filtered water.

4. *Take an electrically formulated herbal cleanse.* Do so preferably first thing in the morning and, if necessary, last thing before going to sleep at night.

5. *Rebuild your gut bacteria.* Repopulate your gut bacteria with live active enzymes and flora such as Latero Flora (B.O.D. strain of bifidus) Digestive Flora, Friendly Flora (*L salivarius, L. plantarium*), and Ultimate Acidophilus.

6. *Support your liver.* Take an electrically formulated liver-support supplement such as Protein Power or TOCO.

7. *MOVE.* Bounce on an electrically tuned rebounder, dance, run, do TaeBo, or engage in other fun activities with plenty of up and down movement to enhance lymphatic drainage. Be creative!

APPENDIX C.

The Soy Report

TRAGEDY AND HYPE
The Third International Soy Symposium

by Sally Fallon and Mary G. Enig, Ph.D.

"Each year, research on the health effects of soy and soybean components seems to increase exponentially . . . Furthermore, research is not just expanding in the primary areas under investigation, such as cancer, heart disease and osteoporosis; new findings suggest that soy has potential benefits that may be more extensive than previously thought." So writes Mark Messina, PhD, General Chairperson of the Third International Soy Symposium, held in Washington, DC, in November of 1999.[1]

For four days, well-funded scientists who were gathered in the nation's capital made presentations to an admiring press and to their sponsors—United Soybean Board, American Soybean Association, Monsanto, Protein Technologies International, Central Soya, Cargill Foods, Personal Products Company, SoyLife, Whitehall-Robins Healthcare and the soybean councils of Illinois, Indiana, Kentucky, Michigan, Minnesota, Nebraska, Ohio and South Dakota.

The symposium marked the apogee of a decade-long marketing campaign to gain consumer acceptance of tofu, soy milk, soy ice cream, soy cheese, soy sausage and soy derivatives, particularly soy isoflavones such as genistein and diadzen, the estrogen-like compounds found in soybeans. It coincided with an FDA decision, announced October 25, to allow a health claim for products "low in saturated fat and cholesterol" that contain 6.25 grams of soy protein per serving. Breakfast cereals, baked goods, convenience food, smoothie mixes and meat substitutes could now be sold with labels touting benefits to cardiovascular health, as long as these products contained one heaping teaspoon of soy protein per 100-gram serving.

MARKETING THE PERFECT FOOD

"Just imagine you could grow the perfect food. This food not only would provide affordable nutrition, but also would be delicious and easy to prepare in a variety of ways. It would be a healthful food, with no saturated fat. In fact, you would be growing a virtual fountain of youth on your back forty." The author is Dean Houghton, writing for *The Furrow*[2], a magazine published in twelve languages by the John Deere tractor company. "This ideal food would help prevent, and perhaps reverse, some of the world's most dreaded diseases. You could grow this miracle crop in a variety of soils and climates. Its cultivation would build up, not deplete, the land . . . this miracle food already exists . . . It's called soy."

Just imagine. Farmers have been imagining . . . and planting more soy. What was once a minor crop, listed in the 1913 USDA handbook not as a food but as an industrial product, now covers 72 million acres of American farmland. Part of this harvest will be used to feed chickens, turkeys, pigs, cows and salmon. Most of the rest will be squeezed to produce oil for margarine, shortenings and salad dressings.

Advances in technology make it possible to produce isolated soy protein from what was once considered a waste product—the defatted, high-protein soy chips—and then transform something that looks and smells terrible into products that can be consumed by human beings. Flavorings, preservatives, sweeteners, emulsifiers and synthetic nutrients have turned soy protein isolate, the food processors' ugly duckling, into a New Age Cinderella.

Lately, this new fairy-tale food has been marketed not so much for her beauty as for her virtues. Early on, products based on soy protein isolate were sold as extenders and meat substitutes, a strategy that failed to produce the requisite consumer demand. The industry changed its approach. "The quickest way to gain product acceptability in the less affluent society," said an industry spokesman, ". . . is to have the product consumed on its own merit in a more affluent society."[3] So soy is now sold to the upscale consumer, not as a cheap poverty food, but as a miracle substance that will prevent heart disease and cancer, whisk away hot flushes, build strong bones and keep us forever young. The competition—meat, milk, cheese, butter and eggs—has been duly demonized by the appropriate government agencies. Soy serves as meat and milk for a new generation of virtuous vegetarians.

Marketing costs money, especially when it needs to be bolstered with "research," but there's plenty of funds available. All soybean producers pay a mandatory assessment of one-half to one per cent of the net market price of soybeans. The total—something like eighty million dollars annually[4]—supports United Soybean's program to "strengthen the position of soybeans in the market place and maintain and expand domestic and foreign markets for uses for soybeans and soybean products." State soybean councils from Maryland, Nebraska, Delaware, Arkansas, Virginia, North Dakota and Michigan provide another two and one-half million dollars yearly for "research."[5] Private companies like Archer Daniels Midland also contribute their share. ADM spent $4.7 million for advertising on "Meet the Press" and $4.3 million on "Face the Nation" during the course of a year.[6] Public relations firms help convert research projects into newspaper articles and advertising copy; law firms lobby for favorable government regulations; IMF money funds soy processing plants in foreign countries; and free trade policies keep soybean abundance flowing to overseas destinations.

The push for more soy has been relentless and global in its reach. Soy protein is now found in most supermarket breads. It is being used to transform "the humble tortilla, Mexico's corn-based staple food, into a protein-fortified 'super-tortilla' that would give a nutritional boost to the nearly 20 million Mexicans who live in extreme poverty.[7]" Advertising for a new soy-enriched loaf from Allied Bakeries in Britain targets menopausal women seeking relief from hot flashes. Sales are running at a quarter of a million loaves per week.[8]

The soy industry hired Norman Robert Associates, a public relations firm, to "get more soy products onto school menus."[9] The USDA responded with a proposal to scrap the 30 percent limit for soy in school lunches. The NuMenu program would allow unlimited use of soy in student meals. With soy added to hamburgers, tacos and lasagna, dieticians can get the total fat content below 30 per cent of calories, thereby conforming to government dictates. "With the soy-enhanced food items, students are receiving better servings of nutrients and less cholesterol and fat."

Soy milk has posted the biggest gains, soaring from $2 million in 1980 to $300 million in the US last year.[10] Recent advances in processing have transformed the gray, thin, bitter, beany-tasting Asian beverage into a product that western consumers will accept—one that tastes like a milk shake, but without the guilt.

Processing miracles, good packaging, massive advertising and a marketing strategy that stresses the products' possible health benefits account for increasing sales to all age groups. For example, reports that soy helps prevent prostate cancer have made soy milk acceptable to middle-aged men. "You don't have to twist the arm of a 55- to 60-year-old guy to get him to try soy milk," says Mark Messina. Michael Milken, former junk bond financier, has helped the industry shed its hippie image with well-publicized efforts to consume 40 grams of soy protein daily. Now it's OK for stockbrokers to eat soy.

America today, tomorrow the world. Soy milk sales are rising in Canada, even though soy milk there costs twice as much as cow's milk. Soybean milk processing plants are sprouting up in places like Kenya.[11] Even China, where soy really is a poverty food and whose people want more meat, not tofu, has opted to build western-style soy factories, rather than develop western grasslands for grazing animals.[12]

Cinderella's Dark Side

The propaganda that has created the soy sales miracle is all the more remarkable because only a few decades ago the soybean was considered unfit to eat—even in Asia. During the Chou Dynasty (1134–246 BC) the soybean was designated one of the five sacred grains, along with barley, wheat, millet and rice. However, the pictograph for the soybean, which dates from earlier times, indicates that it was not first used as a food; for whereas the pictographs for the other four grains show the seed and stem structure of the plant, the pictograph for the soybean emphasises the root structure. Agricultural literature of the period speaks frequently of the soybean and its use in crop rotation. Apparently the soy plant was initially used as a method of fixing nitrogen.[13]

The soybean did not serve as a food until the discovery of fermentation techniques, sometime during the Chou Dynasty. The first soy foods were fermented products like *tempeh, natto, miso* and soy sauce. At a later date, possibly in the 2nd century B.C., Chinese scientists discovered that a puree of cooked soybeans could be precipitated with calcium sulphate or magnesium sulphate (plaster of Paris or Epsom salts) to make a smooth, pale curd—tofu or bean curd. The use of fermented and precipitated soy products soon spread to other parts of the Orient, notably Japan and Indonesia.

The Chinese did not eat unfermented soybeans as they did other legumes such as lentils because the soybean contains large quantities of natural toxins or "antinutrients." First among them are potent enzyme inhibitors that block the action of trypsin and other enzymes needed for protein digestion. These inhibitors are large, tightly-folded proteins that retain their configuration even when heated for long periods of time. They can produce serious gastric distress, reduced protein digestion and chronic deficiencies in amino acid uptake. In test animals, diets high in trypsin inhibitors cause enlargement and pathological conditions of the pancreas, including cancer.[14]

Soybeans also contain hemagglutinin, a clot-promoting substance that causes red blood cells to clump together.

Trypsin inhibitors and hemagglutinin are growth inhibitors—weanling rats fed soy containing these antinutrients fail to grow normally. Growth depressant compounds are deactivated during the process of fermentation, so once the Chinese discovered how to ferment the soybean, they began to incorporate small amounts of soy foods into their diets. In precipitated products, enzyme inhibitors concentrate in the soaking liquid rather than in the curd. Thus in tofu and bean curd, growth depressants are reduced in quantity, but not completely eliminated.

Soy also contains goitrogens—substances that depress thyroid function, a fact that has been known for at least 50 years.

Soybeans are high in phytic acid, present in the bran or hulls of all seeds, a substance that can block the uptake of essential minerals—calcium, magnesium, copper, iron and especially zinc—in the intestinal tract. Although not a household word, phytic acid has been extensively studied—there are literally hundreds of articles on the effects of phytic acid in the current scientific literature. Researchers are in general agreement that grain- and legume-based diets high in phytates contribute to widespread mineral deficiencies in Third world countries.[15] Analysis shows that calcium, magnesium, iron and zinc are present in the plant foods eaten in these areas, but the high phytate content of soy- and grain-based diets prevents their absorption.

The soybean has one of the highest phytate levels of any grain or legume that has been studied[16] and the phytates in soy are highly resistant to normal phytate-reducing techniques, such as long, slow cooking.[17] Only a long period of fermentation will significantly reduce the phytate content of soybeans. When precipitated soy products like tofu are consumed with meat, the mineral blocking effects of the phytates are reduced.[18] The Japanese traditionally eat a small amount of *tofu* or *miso* as part of a mineral-rich fish broth, followed by a serving of meat or fish.

Vegetarians who consume tofu and bean curd as a substitute for meat and dairy products risk severe mineral deficiencies. The results of calcium, magnesium and iron deficiency are well known, those of zinc are less so. Zinc is called the intelligence mineral because it is needed for optimal development and functioning of the brain and nervous system. It plays a role in protein synthesis and collagen formation; it is involved in the blood sugar control mechanism and thus protects against diabetes; it is needed for a healthy reproductive system. Zinc is a key component in numerous vital enzymes and plays a role in the immune system. Phytates found in soy products interfere with zinc absorption more completely than with other minerals.[19] Zinc deficiency can cause a "spacy" feeling that some vegetarians may mistake for the "high" of spiritual enlightenment.

Milk-drinking is given as the reason why second generation Japanese in America grow taller than their native ancestors. Some investigators postulate that the reduced phytate content of the American diet—whatever may be its other deficiencies—is the true explanation, pointing out that both Asian and Western children who do not get enough meat and fish products to counteract the effects of a high phytate diet, frequently suffer rickets, stunting and other growth problems.[20]

SOY PROTEIN ISOLATE

Soy processors have worked hard to get these antinutrients out of the finished product, particularly soy protein isolate (SPI), which is the key ingredient in most soy foods that imitate meat and dairy products, including baby formulas and some brands of soy milk. SPI is not something you can make in your own kitchen. Production takes place in industrial factories where a slurry of soy beans is first mixed with an alkaline solution to remove fiber, then precipitated and separated using an acid wash and finally neutralized in an alkaline solution. Acid washing in aluminium tanks leaches high levels of aluminium into the final product. The resultant curds are spray dried at high temperatures to produce a high protein powder. A final indignity to the original soy bean is high-temperature, high-pressure extrusion processing of soy protein isolate to produce textured vegetable protein (TVP).

Much of the trypsin inhibitor content can be removed through high-temperature processing, but not all. Trypsin inhibitor content of soy protein isolate can vary as much as fivefold.[21] (In rats, even low-level-trypsin-inhibitor SPI feeding results in reduced weight gain compared to controls.[22]) But high-temperature processing has the unfortunate side effect of so denaturing the other proteins in soy that they are rendered largely ineffective.[23] That's why animals on soy feed need lysine supplements for normal growth.

Nitrites, which are potent carcinogens, are formed during spray drying, and a toxin called lysinoalanine is formed during alkaline processing.[24] Numerous artificial flavorings, particularly MSG, are added to soy protein isolate and textured vegetable protein products to mask their strong "beany" taste, and impart the flavor of meat.[25]

In feeding experiments, use of SPI increased requirements for vitamins E, K, D and B12 and created deficiency symptoms of calcium, magnesium, manganese, molybdenum, copper, iron and zinc.[26] Phytic acid remaining in these soy products greatly inhibits zinc and iron absorption; test animals fed SPI develop enlarged organs, particularly the pancreas and thyroid gland, and increased deposition of fatty acids in the liver.[27] Yet soy protein isolate and textured vegetable protein are used extensively in school lunch programs, commercial baked goods, diet beverages and fast food products. They are heavily promoted in Third World countries and form the basis of many food giveaway programs.

In spite of poor results in animal feeding trials, the soy industry has sponsored a number of studies designed to show that soy protein products can be used in *human* diets as a replacement for traditional foods. An example is "Nutritional Quality of Soy Bean Protein Isolates: Studies in Children of Preschool Age" sponsored by the Ralston Purina Company.[28] A group of Central American children suffering from malnutrition was first stabilized and brought into better health by feeding them native foods, including meat and dairy products. Then for a two-week period these traditional foods were replaced by a drink made of soy protein isolate and sugar. All nitrogen taken in and all nitrogen excreted was measured in truly Orwellian fashion—the children were weighed naked every morning and all excrement and vomit gathered up for analysis. The researchers found that the children retained nitrogen and that their growth was "adequate," so the experiment was declared a success. Whether the children were actually healthy on such a diet, or could remain so over a long period, is another matter. The researchers noted that the children vomited "occasionally," usually after finishing a meal; over half suffered from periods of moderate diarrhea; some had upper respiratory infections; and others suffered from rash and fever. It should be noted that the researchers did not *dare* to use soy products to help the children recover from malnutrition, and were obliged to supplement the soy-sugar mixture with nutrients largely absent in soy products, notably vitamins A, D, B12, iron, iodine and zinc.

FDA HEALTH CLAIM

The best marketing strategy for a product that is inherently unhealthy is, of course, a health claim. "The road to FDA approval was long and demanding," writes a soy apologist, "consisting of a detailed review of human clinical data collected from more than 40 scientific studies conducted over the last 20 years. Soy protein was found to be one of the rare foods that had sufficient scientific evidence not only to qualify for an FDA health claim proposal but to ultimately pass the rigorous approval process."[29] The FDA health claim permitted for any food containing 6.25 grams of soy protein is based on the supposition that four such servings, containing a total of 25 grams of soy protein, can offer substantial protection against heart disease.

The "long and demanding" road to FDA approval actually took a few unexpected turns. The original petition, submitted by Protein Technologies International (a division of DuPont), requested a health claim for isoflavones, the estrogen-like compounds found plentifully in soybeans, based on assertions that "only soy protein that has been processed in a manner in which isoflavones are retained will result in cholesterol-lowering." In 1998, the FDA made the unprecedented move of rewriting PTI's petition, removing any reference to the phytoestrogens and substituting a claim for soy protein, a move that was in direct contradiction to the agency's regulations. The FDA is authorized to make rulings only on substances presented by petition.

The abrupt change in direction was no doubt due to the fact that a number of researchers, including scientists employed by the US government, submitted documents indicating that isoflavones are toxic. The FDA had also received, early in 1998, the final British government report on phytoestrogens, which failed to find much evidence of benefit and warned against potential adverse effects.[30]

Even with the change to soy protein isolate, FDA bureaucrats engaged in the "rigorous approval process" were forced to deal nimbly with concerns about mineral blocking effects, enzyme inhibitors, goitrogenicity, endocrine disruption, reproductive problems and increased allergic reactions from consumption of soy products.[31] One of the strongest letters of protest came from Dr. Dan Sheehan and Dr. Daniel Doerge, government researchers at the National Center for Toxicological Research.[32] Their pleas for warning labels were dismissed as unwarranted.

"Sufficient scientific evidence" of soy's cholesterol-lowering properties is drawn largely from a 1995 meta-analysis by Dr. James Anderson, sponsored by Protein Technologies International and published in the *New England Journal of Medicine*.[33] A meta-analysis is a review and summary of the results of many clinical studies on the same subject. Use of meta-analyses to draw general conclusions has come under sharp criticism by members of the scientific community. "Researchers substituting meta-analysis for more rigorous trials risk making faulty assumptions and indulging in creative accounting," says Sir John Scott, President of the Royal Society of New Zealand. "Like is not being lumped with like. Little lumps and big lumps of data are being gathered together by various groups."[34] There is the added temptation for researchers, particularly researchers funded by a company like Protein Technologies International, to leave out studies that would prevent the desired conclusions. Dr. Anderson discarded eight studies for various reasons, leaving a remainder of 29. The published report suggested that individuals with cholesterol levels over 250 mg/dl would experience a "significant" reduction of 7 to 20 percent in levels of serum cholesterol if they substituted soy protein for animal protein. Cholesterol reduction was *insignificant* for individuals whose cholesterol was lower than 250 mg/dl. In other words, for most of us, giving up steak and eating vegeburgers instead will not bring down blood cholesterol levels. The health claim that the FDA approved "after detailed review of human clinical data" fails to inform the consumer about these important details.

Research that ties soy to positive effects on cholesterol levels is "incredibly immature," said Ronald M. Krauss, M.D., head of the Molecular Medical Research Program and Lawrence Berkeley National Laboratory.[35] He might have added that studies in which cholesterol levels were lowered either through diet or drugs have consistently resulted in a greater number of deaths in the treatment groups than in controls, deaths from stroke, cancer, intestinal disorders, accident and suicide.[36] Cholesterol lowering measures in the US have fuelled a sixty-billion-dollar-a-year cholesterol-lowering industry, but have not saved us from the ravages of heart disease.

SOY AND CANCER

The new FDA ruling does not allow any claims about cancer prevention on food packages, but that has not restrained the industry and its marketeers from making them in their promotional literature. "In addition to protecting the heart," says a vitamin company brochure, "soy has demonstrated powerful anticancer benefits . . . the Japanese, who eat 30 times as much soy as North Americans, have a lower incidence of cancers of the breast, uterus and prostate."[37]

Indeed they do. But the Japanese, and Asians in general, have much higher rates of other types of cancer, particularly cancer of the esophagus, stomach, pancreas and liver.[38] Asians throughout the world also have high rates of thyroid cancer.[39] The logic that links low rates of reproductive cancers to soy consumption requires attribution of high rates of thyroid and digestive cancers to the same foods, particularly as soy causes these types of cancers in laboratory rats.

Just how much soy do Asians eat? The famous Cornell China Study, conducted by Colin T. Campbell, found that legume consumption in China varied from 0 to 58 grams per day, with a mean of about 12.[41] Assuming that two-thirds of legume consumption is soy, then the maximum consumption is about 40 grams or less than 3 tablespoons per day, with an average consumption of about 9 grams, less than two teaspoons. A survey conducted in the 1970s found that soy foods accounted for only 1.5 percent of calories in the Chinese diet, compared with 65 percent of calories from pork.[42] (Asians traditionally cooked in lard, not vegetable oil!) In Japan, soy consumption is somewhat higher. A 1998 survey found that the average daily amount of soy consumed in Japan was about 60 grams or ¼ cup.[40] This translates to about 8 grams of soy protein daily (less than two teaspoons), or about one-third the amount now recommended by the FDA.

Traditionally fermented soy products make a delicious, natural seasoning that may supply important nutritional factors in the Asian diet. But except in times of famine, Asians consume soy products only in small amounts as condiments, and not as a replacement for animal foods—with one exception. Celibate monks living in monasteries and leading a vegetarian lifestyle find soy foods quite helpful because they dampen libido.

It was a 1994 meta-analysis by Mark Messina, published in *Nutrition and Cancer,* that fueled speculation on soy's anticarcinogenic properties.[43] Messina noted that in 26 animal studies, 65 percent reported protective effects from soy. He conveniently neglected to include at least one study in which soy feeding caused pancreatic cancer, the 1985 study by Rackis.[44] In the human studies he listed, the results were mixed. A few showed some protective effect but most showed no correlation at all between soy consumption and cancer rates.

". . . the data in this review cannot be used as a basis for claiming that soy intake decreases cancer risk," he concluded. Yet in his subsequent book, *The Simple Soybean and Your Health,* Messina makes just such a claim, recommending 1 cup or 230 grams of soy products per day in his "optimal" diet as a way to prevent cancer.

Thousands of women are now consuming soy in the belief that it protects them against breast cancer. Yet in 1996 researchers found that women consuming soy protein isolate had an increased incidence of epithelial hyperplasia, a condition that presages malignancies.[45] A year later, dietary genistein was found to stimulate breast cells to enter the cell cycle, a discovery that led the study authors to conclude that women should not consume soy products to prevent breast cancer.[46]

Phytoestrogens — Panacea or Poison?

The male species of tropical birds carries the drab plumage of the female at birth and "colors up" at maturity, somewhere between nine and 24 months. In 1991, Richard and Valerie James, bird breeders in Whangerai, New Zealand, purchased a new kind of feed for their birds, one based largely on soy protein.[47] When soy-based feed was used, their birds "colored up" after just a few months. In fact, one bird food manufacturer claimed that this early development was an advantage imparted by the feed. A 1992 ad for Roudybush feed formula showed a picture of the male crimson rosella, an Australian parrot that acquires beautiful red plumage at 18 to 24 months, already brightly colored at 11 weeks old.

Unfortunately, in the ensuing years, there was decreased fertility in the birds with precocious maturation, deformed, stunted and stillborn babies, and premature deaths, especially among females, with the result that the total population in the aviaries went into steady decline. The birds suffered beak and bone deformities, goitre, immune system disorders and pathological aggressive behavior. Autopsy revealed digestive organs in a state of disintegration. The list of problems corresponded with many of the problems the Jameses had encountered in their two children, who had been fed soy-based infant formula.

Startled, aghast, angry . . . the Jameses hired toxicologist Mike Fitzpatrick to investigate further. Dr. Fitzpatrick's literature review uncovered evidence that soy consumption has been linked to numerous disorders, including infertility, increased cancer and infantile leukemia;

and, in studies dating back to the 1950s,[48] that genistein in soy causes endocrine disruption in animals. Dr. Fitzpatrick also analyzed the bird feed and found that it contained high levels of phytoestrogens, especially genistein. When the Jameses discontinued using soy-based feed, the flock gradually returned to normal breeding habits and behavior.

The Jameses embarked on a private crusade to warn the public and government officials about toxins in soy foods, particularly the endocrine-disrupting isoflavones (genistein and diadzen). Protein Technologies International received their material in 1994.

In 1991, Japanese researchers reported that consumption of as little as 30 grams or 2 tablespoons of soybeans per day for only one month resulted in a significant increase in thyroid stimulating hormone.[49] Diffuse goitre and hypothyroidism appeared in some of the subjects and many complained of constipation, fatigue and lethargy, even though their intake of iodine was adequate. In 1997, researchers from the FDA's National Center for Toxicological Research made the embarrassing discovery that the goitrogenic components of soy were the very same isoflavones.[50]

Twenty-five grams of soy protein isolate, the minimum amount PTI claimed to have cholesterol-lowering effects, contains at least 50 mg of isoflavones. It took only 45 mg daily of isoflavones in premenopausal women to exert significant biological effects including reduction in hormones needed for adequate thyroid function. These effects lingered for three months after soy consumption was discontinued.[51]

One hundred grams of soy protein, the maximum suggested cholesterol-lowering dose (and the amount recommended by Protein Technologies International), can contain almost 600 mg of isoflavones,[52] an amount that is undeniably toxic. In 1992, the Swiss health service estimated that 100 grams of soy protein provided the estrogenic equivalent of the pill.[53]

In vitro studies suggest that isoflavones inhibit synthesis of estradiol and other steroid hormones.[54] Reproductive problems, infertility, thyroid disease and liver disease due to dietary intake of isoflavones have been observed for several species of animals including mice, cheetah, quail, pigs, rats, sturgeon and sheep.[55]

It is the isoflavones in soy that are said to have a favorable effect on postmenopausal symptoms, including hot flashes and protection from osteoporosis. Quantification of discomfort from hot flashes is extremely subjective and most studies show that control subjects report reduction in discomfort in amounts equal to subjects given soy.[56]

The claim that soy prevents osteoporosis is extraordinary, given that soy foods block calcium and cause vitamin D deficiencies. If Asians indeed have lower rates of osteoporosis than Westerners, it is because their diet provides plenty of vitamin D from shrimp, lard and seafood, and plenty of calcium from bone broths. The likely reason that Westerners have such high rates of osteoporosis is because they have substituted soy oil for butter, which is a traditional source of vitamin D and other fat-soluble activators needed for calcium absorption.

BIRTH CONTROL PILLS FOR BABIES

But it was the isoflavones in infant formula that gave the Jameses the most cause for concern. In 1998, investigators reported that the daily exposure of infants to isoflavones in soy infant formula is 6 to 11 times higher on a body weight basis than the dose that has hormonal effects in adults consuming soy foods. Circulating concentrations of isoflavones in infants fed soy-based formula were 13,000 to 22,000 times higher than plasma estradiol concentrations in infants on cow's milk formula.[57]

Approximately 25 per cent of bottle-fed children in the US receive soy-based formula—a much higher percentage than in other parts of the Western world. Fitzpatrick estimated that an infant exclusively fed soy formula receives the estrogenic equivalent (based on body weight) of at least five birth control pills per day.[58] By contrast, almost no phytoestrogens have been detected in dairy-based infant formula or in human milk, even when the mother consumes soy products.

Scientists have known for years that soy-based formula can cause thyroid problems in babies. But what are the effects of soy products on the hormonal development of the infant, both male and female?

Male infants undergo a "testosterone surge" during the first few months of life, when testosterone levels may be as high as those of an adult male. During this period, the infant is programmed to express male characteristics after puberty, not only in the development of his sexual organs and other masculine physical traits, but also in setting patterns in the brain characteristic of male behavior. In monkeys, deficiency of male hormones impairs the development of spatial perception (which, in humans, is normally more acute in men than in women), of learning ability and of visual discrimination tasks (such as would be required for reading).[59] It goes without saying that future patterns of sexual orientation may also be influenced by the early hormonal environment. Male children exposed during gestation to diethylstilbestrol (DES), a synthetic estrogen that has effects on animals similar to those of phytoestrogens from soy, had testes smaller than normal on maturation.[60]

Learning disabilities and behavioral problems, especially in male children, have reached epidemic proportions in the U.S. Soy infant feeding—which began in earnest in the early 1970s—cannot be ignored as a probable cause for these tragic developments.

As for girls, an alarming number are entering puberty much earlier than normal, according to a recent study reported in the journal *Pediatrics*.[61] Investigators found that one percent of all girls now show signs of puberty, such as breast development or pubic hair, before the age of three; by age eight, 14.7 percent of white girls and almost 50 percent of African-American girls have one or both of these characteristics. New data indicate that environmental estrogens such as PCBs and DDE (a breakdown product of DDT) may cause early sexual development in girls.[62] In the 1986 Puerto Rico Premature Thelarche study, the most significant dietary association with premature sexual development was not chicken—as reported in the press—but soy infant formula.[63] The Woman, Infants and Children (WIC) program, which supplies free infant formula to welfare mothers, stresses soy formula for African Americans because they are supposedly allergic to milk.

The consequences of this truncated childhood are tragic. Young girls with mature bodies must cope with feelings and urges that most children are not well-equipped to handle. And early maturation in girls is frequently a harbinger for problems with the reproductive system later in life including failure to menstruate, infertility and breast cancer.

Parents who have contacted the Jameses recount other problems associated with children of both sexes who were fed soy-based formula including extreme emotional behavior, asthma, immune system problems, pituitary insufficiency, thyroid disorders and irritable bowel syndrome—the same endocrine and digestive havoc that afflicted the Jameses' parrots.

DISSENTION IN THE RANKS

Organizers of the Third International Soy Symposium would be hard pressed to call the conference an unqualified success. On the second day of the conference, the London-based Food Commission and the Weston A. Price Foundation of Washington, D.C., held a joint press conference in the same hotel to present concerns about soy infant formula. Industry representatives sat stony faced through the recitation of potential dangers and a plea from concerned scientists and parents to pull soy-based infant formula from the market. Under pressure from the Jameses, the New Zealand Government had issued a health warning about soy infant formula in 1998; it was time for the American government to do the same.

On the last day of the conference, presentations on new findings related to toxicity sent a well-oxygenated chill through the giddy helium hype. Dr. Lon White reported on a study of Japanese Americans living in Hawaii. It showed a significant statistical relationship between two or more servings of tofu a week and "accelerated brain aging".[64] Those participants who consumed tofu in mid life had lower cognitive function in late life and a greater incidence of Alzheimers and dementia. "What's more," said Dr. White, "those who ate a lot of tofu, by the time they were 75 or 80, looked five years older."[65] White and his colleagues blamed the negative effects on isoflavones, a finding that supports an earlier study in which post-menopausal women with higher levels of circulating estrogen experienced greater cognitive decline.[66]

Scientists Daniel Sheehan and Daniel Doerge from the National Center for Toxicological Research ruined PTI's day by presenting findings from rat feeding studies indicating that genistein in soy foods causes irreversible damage to enzymes that synthesize thyroid hormones.[67] "The association between soybean consumption and goiter in animals and humans has a long history," wrote Dr. Doerge. "Current evidence for the beneficial effects of soy requires a full understanding of potential adverse effects as well."

Dr. Claude Hughes reported that rats born to mothers fed genistein had decreased birth weights compared to controls and onset of puberty occurred earlier in male offspring.[68] His research suggested that the effects observed in rats ". . . will be at least somewhat predictive of what occurs in humans. There is no reason to assume that there will be gross malformations of fetuses but there may be subtle changes, such as neurobehavioral attributes, immune function and sex hormone levels." The results, he said, ". . . could be nothing or could be something of great concern . . . if mom is eating something that can act like sex hormones, it is logical to wonder if that could change the baby's development."[69]

A study of babies born to vegetarian mothers, published in January 2000, indicated just what those changes in baby's development might be. Mothers who ate a vegetarian diet during pregnancy had a fivefold greater risk of delivering a boy with hypospadias, a birth defect of the penis.[70] The authors of the study suggested that the cause was greater exposure to phytoestrogens in soy foods popular with vegetarians. Problems with female offspring of vegetarian mothers are more likely to show up later in life. While soy's estrogenic effect is less than that of diethylstilbestrol (DES), the dose is likely to be higher because it's consumed as a food, not taken as a drug. Daughters of women who took DES during pregnancy suffered from infertility and cancer when they reached their twenties.

GRAS STATUS

Lurking in the background of industry hoop-la for soy is the nagging question of whether it's even legal to add soy protein isolate to food. All food additives not in common use prior to 1958, including casein protein from milk, must have GRAS (Generally Recognized As Safe) status. In 1972, the Nixon administration directed a reexamination of substances believed to be GRAS in the light of any scientific information then available. This reexamination included casein protein which became codified as GRAS in 1978. In 1974, the FDA obtained a literature review of soy protein because, as soy protein had not been used in food until 1959 and was not even in common use in the early 1970s, it was not eligible to have its GRAS status grandfathered under the provisions of the Food, Drug and Cosmetic Act.[71]

The scientific literature up to 1974 recognized many antinutrients in factory-made soy protein, including trypsin inhibitors, phytic acid and genistein. But the FDA literature review dismissed discussion of adverse impacts with the statement that it was important for "adequate processing" to remove them. Genistein could be removed with an alcohol wash but it was an expensive procedure that processors avoided. Later studies determined that trypsin inhibitor content could be removed only with long periods of heat and pressure, but the FDA has imposed no requirements for manufacturers to do so.

The FDA was more concerned with toxins formed during processing, specifically nitrites and lysinoalanine.[72] Even at low levels of consumption—averaging one-third of a gram per day at the time—the presence of these carcinogens was considered too great a threat to public health to allow GRAS status. Soy protein did have approval for use as a binder in cardboard boxes and this approval was allowed to continue because researchers considered that migration of nitrites from the box into the food contents would be too small to constitute a cancer risk. FDA officials called for safety specifications and monitoring procedures before granting of GRAS status for food. These were never performed. To this day, use of soy protein is codified as GRAS only for this limited industrial use as a cardboard binder.

This means that soy protein must be subject to premarket approval procedures each time manufacturers intend to use it as a food or add it to a food. Soy protein was introduced into infant formula in the early 1960s. It was a new product with no history of any use at all. As soy protein did not have GRAS status, premarket approval was required. This was not and still has not been granted. The key ingredient of soy infant formula is not recognized as safe.

THE NEXT ASBESTOS?

"Against the backdrop of widespread praise . . . there is growing suspicion that soy—despite its undisputed benefits—may pose some health hazards," writes Marian Burros, a leading food writer for the *New York Times*. More than any other writer, Ms. Burros's endorsement of a low-fat, largely vegetarian diet has herded Americans into supermarket aisles featuring soy foods. Yet her January 26, 2000 article, "Doubts Cloud Rosy News on Soy" contains the following alarming statement: "Not one of the 18 scientists interviewed for this column was willing to say that taking isoflavones was risk free." Ms. Burros did not enumerate the risks, nor did she mention that the recommended 25 daily grams of soy protein contain enough isoflavones to cause problems in sensitive individuals, but it was evident that the industry had recognized the need to cover itself.

Because the industry is extremely exposed, contingency lawyers will soon discover that the number of potential plaintiffs can be counted in the millions and the pockets are very, very deep. Juries will hear something like the following: "The industry has known for years that soy contains many toxins. At first they told the public that the toxins were removed by processing. When it became apparent that processing could not get rid of them, they claimed that these substances were beneficial. Your government granted a health claim to a substance that is poisonous and the industry lied to the public to sell more soy."

The "industry" includes merchants, manufacturers, scientists, publicists, bureaucrats, former bond financiers, food writers, vitamin companies and retail stores. Farmers will probably escape because they were duped like the rest of us. But they need to find something else to grow before the soy bubble bursts and the market collapses—grass-fed livestock, designer vegetables . . . or hemp to make paper for thousands and thousands of legal briefs.

Sally Fallon is the author of *Nourishing Traditions: The Cookbook that Challenges Politically Correct Nutrition and the Diet Dictocrats*, Second Edition 1999 (New Trends Publishing 877-707-1776 or 219-268-2601) and President of the Weston A Price Foundation, Washington, D.C., www.WestonAPrice.org

Mary G. Enig, Ph.D., is the author of *Know Your Fats: The Complete Primer for Understanding the Nutrition of Fats, Oils and Cholesterol* 2000 (www.BethesdaPress.com), President of the Maryland Nutritionists Association and Vice President of the Weston A Price Foundation, Washington, D.C.

The authors wish to thank Mike Fitzpatrick, Ph.D., and Valerie & Richard James for their help in preparing this article.

NOTES

1. Program for the Third International Symposium on the *Role of Soy in Preventing and Treating Chronic Disease*, Sunday, October 31, through Wednesday, November 3, 1999, Omni Shoreham Hotel, Washington, DC.
2. Dean Houghton, "Healthful Harvest," *The Furrow*, January 2000, pp. 10–13.
3. Richard J Coleman, "Vegetable Protein—A Delayed Birth?" *Journal of the American Oil Chemists' Society*, April 1975, 52:238A.
4. See http://www/unitedsoybean.org.
5. These are listed in www.soyonlineservice.co.nz.
6. *Wall Street Journal*, October 27, 1995.
7. James F Smith, "Healthier tortillas could lead to healthier Mexico," *The Denver Post*, August 22, 1999, p. 26A.
8. "Bakery says new loaf can help reduce hot flushes," *Reuters*, September 15, 1997.
9. "Beefing Up Burgers with Soy Products at School," *Nutrition Week*, Community Nutrition Institute, Washington, DC, June 5, 1998, p. 2.
10. John Urquhart, "A Health Food Hits Big Time," *Wall Street Journal*, August 3, 1999, p. B1
11. "Soyabean Milk Plant in Kenya," *Africa News Service*, September 1998.
12. Frederick J Simoons, *Food in China: A Cultural and Historical Inquiry*, CRC Press, Boca Raton, 1991, page 64.
13. Solomon H Katz, "Food and Biocultural Evolution: A Model for the Investigation of Modern Nutritional Problems," *Nutritional Anthropology*, Alan R. Liss Inc., 1987, page 50.
14. Joseph J Rackis, et al, "The USDA trypsin inhibitor study. I. Background, objectives and procedural details," *Qualification of Plant Foods in Human Nutrition*, 1985, volume 35.
15. Van-Rensburg et al, "Nutritional status of African populations predisposed to esophageal cancer," *Nutrition and Cancer*, 1983 4:206–216; P B Moser, et al, "Copper, iron, zinc and sele-

nium dietary intake and status of Nepalese lactating women and their breast-fed infants," *American Journal of Clinical Nutrition*, April 1988, 47:729–734; B F Harland, et al, "Nutritional status and phytate: zinc and phytate X calcium: zinc dietary molar ratios of lacto-ovo-vegetarian Trappist monks: 10 years later," *Journal of the American Dietetic Association*, December 1988, 88:1562–1566.

16. A H El Tiney, "Proximate Composition and Mineral and Phytate Contents of Legumes Grown in Sudan," *Journal of Food Composition and Analysis*, 1989, 2:67–68.

17. A D Ologhobo, et al, "Distribution of phosphorus and phytate in some Nigerian varieties of legumes and some effects of processing," *Journal of Food Science*, January/February 1984, 49(1):199–201.

18. B Sandstrom, et al, "Effect of protein level and protein source on zinc absorption in humans," *Journal of Nutrition*, January 1989, 119(1):48–53; Susan Tait, et al, "The availability of minerals in food, with particular reference to iron," *Journal of Research in Society and Health*, April 1983, 103(2):74–77.

19. Phytate reduction of zinc absorption has been demonstrated in numerous studies. These results are summarized in Richard Leviton, *Tofu, Tempeh Miso and Other Soyfoods: The "Food of the Future"—How to Enjoy Its Spectacular Health Benefits*, Keats Publishing, Inc., New Canaan, CT 1982, pages 14–15.

20. Edward Mellanby, "Experimental rickets: The effect of cereals and their interaction with other factors of diet and environment in producing rickets," *Journal of the Medical Research Council*, March 1925 93:265; M R Wills, et al, "Phytic Acid and Nutritional Rickets in Immigrants," *The Lancet*, April 8,1972, pages 771–773.

21. Joseph J Rackis, et al, "The USDA trypsin inhibitor study. I. Background, objectives and procedural details," *Qualification of Plant Foods in Human Nutrition*, 1985, volume 35

22. Joseph J Rackis, et al, "The USDA trypsin inhibitor study. I. Background, objectives and procedural details," *Qualification of Plant Foods in Human Nutrition*, 1985, volume 35:232.

23. Wallace, G.M., "Studies on the Processing and Properties of Soymilk," *Journal of Science and Food Agriculture*, October 1971, 22:526–535.

24. Joseph Rackis, et al, "The USDA trypsin inhibitor study. I. Background, objectives and procedural details," *Qualification of Plant Foods in Human Nutrition*, 1985, volume 35:22; "Evaluation of the Health Aspects of Soy Protein Isolates as Food Ingredients," Prepared for FDA by Life Sciences Research Office, *Federation of American Societies for Experimental Biology*, 9650 Rockville Pike, Bethesda, MD 20014, Contract No, FDA 223-75-2004, 1979.

25. See http://www/truthinlabeling.org.

26. Joseph J Rackis, "Biological and physiological Factors in Soybeans," *Journal of the American Oil Chemists' Society*, January 1974, 51:161A-170A.

27. Joseph J Rackis, et al, "The USDA trypsin inhibitor study. I. Background, objectives and procedural details," *Qualification of Plant Foods in Human Nutrition*, 1985, volume 35

28. Benjamin Torum, "Nutritional Quality of Soybean Protein Isolates: Studies in Children of Preschool Age," in *Soy Protein and Human Nutrition*, Harold L Wilcke et al, eds, Academic Press, New York, 1979.

29. Marwin Zreik, CCN, "The Great Soy Protein Awakening," *Total Health*, February 2000, Vol 32, No 1.

30. *IEH assessment on Phytoestrogens in the Human Diet*, Final Report to the Ministry of Agriculture, Fisheries and Food, UK, November 1997, page 11.

31. *Food Labeling: Health Claims: Soy Protein and Coronary Heart Disease*, Food and Drug Administration 21 CFR Part 101 (Docket No. 98P-0683).

32. Daniel M Sheegan and Daniel R Doerge, Letter to Dockets Management Branch (HFA-305), February 18, 1999.

33. James W Anderson, et al, "Meta-analysis of the Effects of Soy Protein Intake on Serum Lipids," *New England Journal of Medicine*, 1995 333:(5):276–82.

34. Camille Guy, "Doctors warned against magic, quackery," *New Zealand Herald*, September 9, 1995, Section Eight, Page 5.

35. Kate Sander and Hilary Wilson, "FDA approves new health claim for soy, but litte fallout expected for dairy," *Cheese Market News*, October 22, 1999, page 24.

36. Mary G Enig, and Sally Fallon, "The Oiling of America," *Nexus Magazine*, December 1998–January 1999 and February 1999–March 1999, also available at www.WestonAPrice.org.

37. "Natural Medicine News," L & H Vitamins, 32–33 47th Avenue, Long Island City, NY 11101, January/February 2000, page 8.

38. Angela Harras, Ed. *Cancer Rates and Risks*, 4th Edition, 1996, National Institutes of Health, National Cancer Institute.

39. Charles E Searle, Ed, *Chemical Carcinogens*, ACS Monograph 173, American Chemical Society, Washington, DC, 1976.

40. T Colin Campbell, et al, *The Cornell Project in China*

41. K C Chang, ed, *Food in Chinese Culture: Anthropological and Historical Perspectives*, New Haven, 1977.

42. C Nagata, et al, *Journal of Nutrition*, 1998, 128:209–13.

43. Mark J Messina, et al, "Soy Intake and Cancer Risk: A Review of the In Vitro and In Vivo Data," *Nutrition and Cancer*, 1994, 21(2):113–131.

44. Joseph J Rackis, et al, "The USDA trypsin inhibitor study. I. Background, objectives and procedural details," *Qualification of Plant Foods in Human Nutrition*, 1985, volume 35

45. N L Petrakis, et al, "Stimulatory influence of soy protein isolate on breast secretion in pre- and postmenopausal women," *Cancer Epid Bio Prev* 1996 5:785–794.

46. C Dees, et al, "Dietary estrogens stimulate human breast cells to enter the cell cycle," *Environmental Health Perspectives* 1997, 105(Suppl 3):633–636.

47. D J Woodhams, "Phytoestrogens and parrots: The anatomy of an investigation," *Proceedings of the Nutrition Society of New Zealand*, 1995, 20:22–30.

48. G Matrone et al, "Effect of Genistin on Growth and Development of the Male Mouse," *Journal of Nutrition*, 1956, 235–240.

49. Y Ishizuki, et al, "The effects on the thyroid gland of soybeans administered experimentally in healthy subjects," *Nippon Naibunpi Gakkai Zasshi* 1991, 767:622–629.

50. R L Divi, et al, "Anti-thyroid isoflavones from the soybean," *Biochemical Pharmacology*, 1997, 54:1087–1096.

51. A Cassidy, et al, "Biological Effects of a Diet of Soy Protein Rich in Isoflavones on the Menstrual Cycle of Premenopausal Women," *American Journal of Clinical Nutrition* 1994 60:333–340 (1994).

52. P A Murphy, "Phytoestrogen Content of Processed Soybean Foods," *Food Technology*, 1982, pages 50–54.

53. *Bulletin de L'Office Federal de la Sante Publique*, No. 28, July 20, 1992.

54. W M Keung, "Dietary estrogenic isoflavones are potent inhibitors of B-hydroxysteroid dehydrogenase of *P testosteronii*," *Biochemical and Biophysical Research Committee* 1995, 215:1137–1144; S I Makela, et al, "Estrogen specific 12 B-hydroxysteroid oxidoreductase type 1 (E.C. 1.1.1.62) as a possible target for the action of phytoestrogens," *PSEBM*, 1995, 208:51–59.

55. K D R Setchell, et al, "Dietary estrogens—a probable cause of infertility and liver disease in captive cheetahs," *Gastroenterology* 93:225–233 (1987); A S Leopald, "Phytoestrogens: Adverse effects on reproduction in California Quail," *Science*, 1976, 191:98–100; Drane H M, et al, "Oestrogenic activity of soya-bean products," *Food Cosmetics and Technology*, 1980, 18:425–427; S Kimura, et al, "Development of malignant goiter by defatted soybean with iodine-free diet in rats," *Gann*, 1976, 67:763–765; C Pelissero, et al, "Estrogenic effect of dietary soybean meal on vitellogenesis in cultured Siberian Sturgeon *Acipenser baeri*," *Gen Comp End* 83:447–457; Braden et al, "The oestrogenic activity and metabolism of certain isoflavones in sheep," *Australian Journal of Agricultural Research* 1967 18:335–348.

56. Jean Ginsburg and Giordana M Prelevic, "Is there a proven place for phytoestrogens in the menopause?" *Climacteric*, 1999, 2:75–78.

57. K D Setchell, et al, "Isoflavone content of infant formulas and the metabolic fate of these early phytoestrogens in early life," *American Journal of Clinical Nutrition*, December 1998, Supplement 1453S–1461S.

58. C Irvine, et al, "The Potential Adverse Effects of Soybean Phytoestrogens in Infant Feeding," *New Zealand Medical Journal*, May 24, 1995, page 318.

59. C Hagger and J Bachevalier, "Visual habit formation in 3-month-old monkeys (Macaca mulatta): reversal of sex difference following neonatal manipulations of androgen," *Behavior and Brain Research* 1991, 45:57–63.

60. R K Ross, et al, "Effect of in-utero exposure to diethylstilbestrol on age at onset of puberty and on post-pubertal hormone levels in boys," *Canadian Medical Association Journal*, May 15, 1983, 128(10):1197–8.

61. Marcia E Herman-Giddens, et al, "Secondary Sexual Characteristics and Menses in Young Girls Seen in Office Practice: A Study from the Pediatric Research in Office Settings Network," *Pediatrics*, April 1997, 99(4):505–512.

62. *Rachel's Environment & Health Weekly*, #263, The Wingspread Statement, Part 1, December 11, 1991; Theo Colborn, Dianne Dumanoski and John Peterson Myers, *Our Stolen Future*, Little Brown and Company, London, 1996.

63. L W Freni-Titulaer, "Premature Thelarch in Puerto Rico, A search for environmental factors," *American Journal of Diseases of Children*, December 1986, 140(12):1263–1267.

64. Lon White, "Association of High Midlife Tofu Consumption with Accelerated Brain Aging," Plenary Session #8: Cognitive Function, The Third International Soy Symposium, Program, November 1999, page 26.

65. Helen Altonn, "Too much tofu induces 'brain aging,' study shows," *Honolulu Star-Bulletin*, November 19, 1999.

66. *Journal of the American Geriatric Society*, 1998, 46:816–21.

67. Daniel R Doerge, "Inactivation of Thyroid Peroxidase by Genistein and Daidzein in Vitro and in Vivo; Mechanism for Anti-Thyroid Activity of Soy," presented at the November, 1999 Soy Symposium in Washington, DC National Center for Toxicological Research, Jefferson, AR 72029.

68. Claude Hughes, Center for Women's Health and Department of Obstetrics & Gynecology, Cedars-Sinai Medical Center, Los Angeles, CA.

69. Soy Intake May Affect Fetus," *Reuters News Service*, November 5, 1999.

70. "Vegetarian diet in pregnancy linked to birth defect," *British Journal of Urology International*, January 2000, 85:107–113.

71. FDA ref 72/104, Report FDABF GRAS—258.

72. "Evaluation of the Health Aspects of Soy Protein Isolates as Food Ingredients," Prepared for FDA by Life Sciences Research Office, *Federation of American Societies for Experimental Biology*, 9650 Rockville Pike, Bethesda, MD 20014, Contract No, FDA 223-75-2004, 1979.

Endnotes

CHAPTER 1

1. Lazarou, J.; B. H. Pomeranz; and P. N. Corey, "Incidence of adverse drug reactions in hospitalized patients: a meta-analysis of prospective studies." *Journal of the American Medical Association* 279 (1998): 1200–1205.

2. Johnson, Jeffrey A., and J. Lyle Bootman, "Drug-related morbidity and mortality." *Archives of Internal Medicine* 155 (October 9, 1995): 1949–1956.

CHAPTER 3

1. Emoto, Masaru. *The Message from Water*, (Tokyo: HADO, 2000).

2. Byrnes, Stephen, "The Other Side of Vegetarianism." *Health and Healing Wisdom* 24(2): 29.

3. Price, Weston. *Nutrition and Physical Degeneration* (New Canaan, CT: Keats Publishing, 1998).

4. Draper, H. H. *Nutrition Studies: The Aboriginal Eskimo Diet—A Modern Perspective* (Stroudsburg, PA: Dowden, Hutchinson, & Ross, Inc., 1978).

5. Stefansson, Vilhjalmur. "Food and food habits in Alaska and Northern Canada." In *Human Nutrition, Historic and Scientific*, ed. Iago Galdston (New York: International University Press, Inc., 1960): 23–60.

6. Pottinger, Jr., Francis M, "The effect of heat-processed foods and metabolized vitamin D milk on the dentofacial structures of experimental animals." *American Journal of Orthodontics and Oral Surgery* 32 (8) (Aug. 1946): 467–485.

7. Dalai Lama. *Freedom from Exile: The Autobiography of the Dalai Lama* (San Francisco: Harper & Row, 1991).

CHAPTER 4

1. U.S. Senate Document 264, 1936, 74th Congress, 2nd session, AD1936USA.

2. Spindler, Conrad. *The Man in the Ice: The Discovery of a 5,000-Year-Old Body Reveals Secrets of the Stone Age* (Toronto: Doubleday, 1994).

CHAPTER 5

1. Hood, V. L., and R. L. Tannen, "Mechanisms of disease: protection of acid-base balance by pH regulation of acid production." *New England Journal of Medicine* 339 (Sept. 17, 1998): 819–826.

2. L. Markowitz; S. Preblud; W. Orenstein; et al., "Patterns of transmission in measles outbreaks in the United States, 1985–1986." *New England Journal of Medicine* 320 (Jan. 12, 1989): 75–81.

3. Classen, J. Barthelow, "Childhood immunisation and diabetes mellitus." *New Zealand Medical Journal*, May 25, 1996, 195.

4. Torch, W. C. "Diphtheria-pertussis-tetanus (DPT) Immunization: A potential cause of the sudden infant death syndrome (SIDS)," (paper presented at the 34th annual meeting of the American Academy of Neurology, April 25–May 1, 1982), 32(4):pt. 2.

5. Dept. of Pediatrics, Georgetown University Medical Center, Washington, DC, "Measles vaccine failures: lack of sustained measles specific immunoglubulin G responses in revaccinated adolescents and young adults." *Pediatric Infectious Disease Journal* 1 (Jan. 1994): 34–38.

6. Div. of Field Epidemiology, Centers for Disease Control and Prevention, Atlanta, "Sustained transmission of mumps in a highly vaccinated population: assessment of primary vaccine failure and waning vaccine-induced immunity." *Journal of Infectious Diseases* 169 (1) (Jan. 1, 1994): 77–82.

7. Dept. of Internal Medicine, Mayo Vaccine Research Group, Mayo Clinic and Foundation, "Apparent paradox of measles infections in immunized persons" (review article: 50 REFS), *Archives of Internal Medicine.* 154(16) (Aug. 1994): 1815–1820.

8. Gunn, Trevor, "Mass immunization: a point in question." In *Pasteur Exposed—The False Foundations of Modern Medicine,* ed. Hume (Australia: Bookreal, 1989), 15.

9. R. W. Sutter; P. A. Patriarca; S. Brogan; et al., "Outbreak of paralytic poliomyelitis in Oman; evidence for widespread transmission among fully vaccinated children." *Lancet* 338 (Sept. 21, 1991): 715–720.

10. www.medical-library.net/sites/_vaccinations.html

11. Collier, Richard. *The Plague of the Spanish Lady* (New York: Atheneum, 1974) 305.

12. Health Resources and Services Administration, *VICP Monthly Statistics Report,* through April 30, 2001: www.bhpr.hrsa.gov/vicp/monthly.html

13. Fulginiti, Vincent A., M.D., and Ray E. Helfer, M.D. "Atypical measles in adolescent siblings 16 years after killed measles virus vaccine." *JAMA* 244 (1980): 804–806.

14. Armstrong, Natalie, "Girl's death accelerates meningitis vaccine plan," *Vancouver Sun,* Jan. 2, 1998.

15. Epstein, Samuel S., M.D. *The Politics of Cancer Revisited* (NY: East Ridge Press, 1998).

16. Moss, Ralph W. *Questioning Chemotherapy* (Brooklyn: Equinox Press, 1995).

17. European Court of Human Rights, *Swiss Association of Electroapparatuses (FEA)* vs. *Hertel,* August 25, 1998. *Journal of Natural Science* 2, (3) (Jan.–Apr. 1999).

18. Roberts, H. J. *Aspartame: Is It Safe?* (Philadelphia: The Charles Press, 1989).

19. Blaycock, Russell L. *Excitotoxins: The Taste that Kills,* (Santa Fe, NM: Health Press, 1996).

20. Maher, Timothy J., Richard Wurtman. "Possible Neurologic Effects of Aspartame, a Widely Used Additive," *Environmental Health Perspectives* 75 (1987): 53–57.

21. www.dorway.com

22. *Congressional Record,* Aug. 1, 1985, SID835.

23. Roberts, H. J. "Reactions Attributed to Aspartame-Containing Products: 551 Cases," *Journal of Applied Nutrition* 40 (1988) 85–94.

24. Wurtman, Richard J. "Aspartame: Possible Effect on Seizure Susceptibility," *The Lancet* 2 (1985): 1060.

25. Walton, Ralph G. "Seizure and Mania after High Intake of Aspartame," *Psychomatics* 27 (1986): 218–222.

26. Walton, Ralph G. "The Possible Role of Aspartame in Seizure Induction." Proceedings of the First International Meeting on Dietary Phenylalanine and Brain Function, Washington, D.C., May 8–10, 1987.

CHAPTER 6

1. Jensen, Bernard. *Come Alive* (Escondido, CA: Self-published, 1997).

CHAPTER 7

1. Mokdad, Ali H.; Mary K Serdula; William H. Dietz; et al., "The Spread of the Obesity Epidemic in the United States 1991–1998." *JAMA* 282 (Oct. 27, 1999): 1519–1522.

2. Stein, Joel, "The Low-Carb Diet Craze." *Time* 154 (18) (Nov. 1999): 75.

CHAPTER 8

1. Robbins, John; Marriane Williamson; and H. J. Kramer. Reclaiming our health: exploding the medical myth and embracing the sources of true healing (Novato, CA: New World Library, 1998).

2. Semmelweiss, Ignaz. *The Etiology, Concept, and Prophylaxis of Childbed Fever,* trans. and ed. K. Codell Carter (Madison: Univ. of Wisconsin Press, 1983).

Index

About the Authors

Denie and Shelley Hiestand are the founders of the International Institute of Vibrational Wellness, which teaches health, personal growth, awareness, and vibrational medicine seminars in the United States, Canada, the United Kingdom, Switzerland, and New Zealand. Known as the "body electrician," Denie is a natural health consultant and the author of the autobiographical *Journey to Truth*. The Hiestands live and practice in Marina del Rey, California. Visit their website at www.vibrationalmedicine.com.